T0201367

Breed Predispositions to Dental and Oral Disease in Dogs

Breed Predispositions to Dental and Oral Disease in Dogs

Edited by
Brook A. Niemiec, DVM, DAVDC, DEVDC, FAVD
Veterinary Dental Specialties and Oral Surgery
San Diego, CA, USA

WILEY Blackwell

Registered Office
John Wiley & Sons, Inc., 111 River Street, Hoboken, NJ 07030, USA

Editorial Office
111 River Street, Hoboken, NJ 07030, USA

For details of our global editorial offices, customer services, and more information about Wiley products visit us at www.wiley.com.

Wiley also publishes its books in a variety of electronic formats and by print-on-demand. Some content that appears in standard print versions of this book may not be available in other formats.

Library of Congress Cataloging-in-Publication Data

Names: Niemiec, Brook A., editor.
Title: Breed predispositions to dental and oral disease in dogs / edited by Brook Niemiec.
Description: Hoboken, NJ : Wiley-Blackwell, 2021. | Includes index.
Identifiers: LCCN 2020024174 (print) | LCCN 2020024175 (ebook) | ISBN 9781119552116 (hardback) | ISBN 9781119552123 (adobe pdf) | ISBN 9781119552048 (epub)
Subjects: MESH: Tooth Diseases–veterinary | Anesthesia, Dental–veterinary | Veterinary Medicine | Dogs
Classification: LCC SF867 (print) | LCC SF867 (ebook) | NLM SF 867 | DDC 636.089/763–dc23
LC record available at https://lccn.loc.gov/2020024174
LC ebook record available at https://lccn.loc.gov/2020024175

Cover Design: Wiley
Cover Images: French bull dog – Robert Furman, Dog dentistry images – Brook A. Niemiec, Blueprint background © belterz /Getty Images

Set in 9.5/12.5pt STIXTwoText by SPi Global, Chennai, India
Printed in Singapore

M094371_260221

Contents

Contributors

Sean W. Aiken, DVM, MS, DACVS
Veterinary Specialty Hospital
San Diego, CA
USA

Amber Hopkins, DVM, cVMA, CCRT,
DACVAA
VCA Alameda East Veterinary Hospital
Denver, CO
USA

Kymberley C. McLeod, DVM
Conundrum Consulting
Toronto, Ontario,
Canada

Brook A. Niemiec, DVM, DAVDC, DEVDC,
FAVD
Veterinary Dental Specialties and Oral Surgery
San Diego, CA
USA

Introduction

Throughout the history of veterinary medicine, when a new species or breed becomes a common focus of therapy, the tendency has been to treat it similarly to historically established methods. These methods serve as a basic guide for therapy, but eventually they are found to be lacking and the profession is required to change its mindset. Thus, the old adages "Dogs are not small horses," and then "Cats are not small dogs."

Veterinary education typically evolves relatively slowly compared to the change in practice demands. Therefore, education may be based on classic models as opposed to what is currently present within daily practice.

With the increasing popularity of "designer" dogs, as well as line breeding for desired traits, we have created hereditable issues within species and breeds. This is perhaps best known and discussed in brachycephalic breeds, but is seen throughout the canine spectrum.

One trend that has been present for decades but is increasing even more rapidly today is the desire for smaller and smaller dogs. These "microdogs" are significantly different in their skeletal as well as behavioral aspects. Perhaps there is nowhere this more apparent than within the oral cavity.

Despite significant differences in the incidence and severity of periodontal disease, we still treat small breed dogs like their larger cousins. This book will describe the significant differences between large and small breed patients in regards to onset, prevalence, and significant local/regional and systemic consequences of periodontal disease. This necessitates a completely different approach to periodontal therapy as well as a reevaluation as to decisions on when and how to extract teeth. We will also cover the other breeds who are prone to particular dental issues and how to mitigate them. In addition, we will briefly cover the unique concerns of brachycephalic breeds. The challenges of extractions in small and toy breed dogs is presented to help avoid iatrogenic complications. Chapters on the animal welfare aspects of heritable oral and dental diseases are included to provide a animal centric, whole patient approach to dental care. Finally, this book will debunk the common myths of anesthetic risks in brachycephalic and especially small breed dogs.

1

Conditions Common in Small and Toy Breed Dogs

Brook A. Niemiec

Veterinary Dental Specialties and Oral Surgery, San Diego, CA, USA

1.1 Periodontal Disease

1.1.1 Periodontal Disease Pathogenesis and Prevalence

Periodontal disease is the most common medical condition in small animal veterinary patients [1, 2]. The classic study from the 1980s reported that by just two years of age, 80% of dogs and 70% of cats have some form of periodontal disease [3]. However, more current studies report that periodontal disease is actually even more common, being diagnosed in 90% of patients by just one year of age [4]. In fact, two studies (one using a sensitive diagnostic test and the other including exam under general anesthesia) revealed that ALL patients in the study were infected [5, 6]. The lack of recognition of the high prevalence of periodontal disease has as much to do with a lack of understanding of the initial signs of disease as it does with the lack of effective diagnostic methods. Part of the issue with diagnosing the early stages of gum disease is that it requires anesthesia (or at least heavy sedation). This is because probing is required (see below) as well as the fact that the earliest signs of disease are typically on the palatal/lingual aspect of the teeth [6].

The earlier onset of periodontal disease is due primarily to the popularity of small and toy breed dogs, who are particularly susceptible [7–11]. The complete reasoning behind this is unknown; however decreased interdental space (crowding) (Figure 1.1) [12], rotation of teeth (Figure 1.2), decreased oral activity (recreational chewing), increased lifespan [13, 14], and shorter tooth roots (Figure 1.3) all likely play a role [15, 16].

There are several additional reasons for the "apparent" increase in incidence. First, the widely known studies from the 1980s were based on erythema of the gingiva being the first sign of gum disease (Figure 1.4). This inflammation is termed "marginal gingivitis" [17, 18], and is created by the proliferation of capillaries and formation of "capillary loops" [19]. While color change is a dependable sign of the presence of gingivitis, it has been established that gingival bleeding on periodontal probing or brushing actually occurs BEFORE any color change [17, 20] (Figure 1.5). Therefore, with new diagnostic tests such as a periodontal diagnostic strip[1], we are finding even more patients affected with periodontal disease. Another reason is the steadily increasing life expectancy in our patients [21, 22]. Small breed dogs are known to live longer than large breeds [13, 14]. This longevity

---

1 Orastrip, PDX biotech

Breed Predispositions to Dental and Oral Disease in Dogs, First Edition. Edited by Brook A. Niemiec.
© 2021 John Wiley & Sons, Inc. Published 2021 by John Wiley & Sons, Inc.

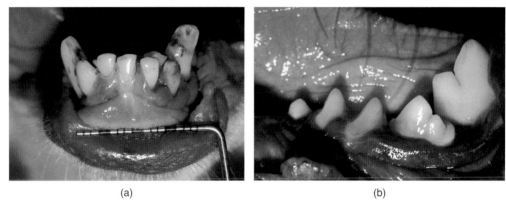

(a)   (b)

Figure 1.1 Crowding. The smaller mouths with relatively larger teeth seen in small and toy breed dogs often results in crowding. Crowding hastens periodontal disease by interfering with the patient's natural cleaning ability as well as the loss of the normal gingival collar. This is demonstrated in the incisor region of a Chihuahua (a) and the mandibular premolar region of a pug (b). Note the periodontal loss on the left side of the patient in (a) as opposed to the more normal right side.

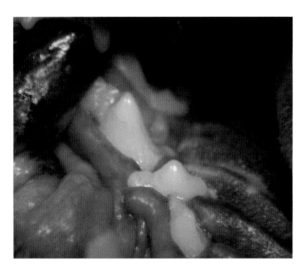

Figure 1.2 Rotated teeth. A rotated maxillary left third premolar (207) of a French Bulldog. Note the lack of spacing between the teeth as well as loss of the gingival collar on both the mesial and distal aspects of this tooth.

provides periodontal disease more time to negatively affect the patient, as it is well known that periodontal disease becomes more common with increasing age [9, 23].

The main factor for the increased susceptibility in certain breeds may also be hereditary in nature. A recent study on Labrador Retrievers revealed that in one litter of eight dogs only 12.5% developed periodontitis, whereas in another litter of five dogs, 100% developed periodontitis [6]. Reports on Schnauzers and Yorkshire Terriers confirmed their propensity to this disease process as well [11, 24, 25]. There are other well known "at risk" breeds besides small and toy breeds (e.g. Greyhounds and Cavalier King Charles Spaniels) [26]. Further, there is mounting research on the human side that there is a genetic predisposition to periodontal disease. Studies on twins showed a significant increase in periodontal disease, attachment loss, and plaque accumulation [27, 28]. Early-onset periodontal disease is ten times more likely to occur in African-Americans when

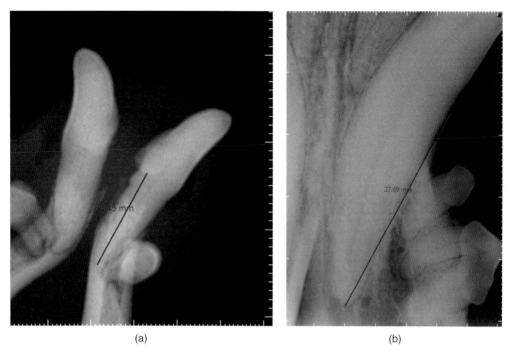

(a)   (b)

Figure 1.3 Root length is significantly reduced in small breed dogs. (a) An intraoral dental radiograph of the mandibular canines of a 0.9 kg Chihuahua. The root length as measured from the cemento-enamel junction (CEJ) to the apex of the root is 8.45 mm. Note that there is also significant alveolar bone loss. (b) An intraoral dental radiograph of the mandibular canines of a 35 kg Labrador Retriever. The root length as measured from the cemento-enamel junction (CEJ) to the apex of the root is 27.69 mm. This means that the roots of the canines are more than three times the length of the same teeth in a small breed dog, thus providing significantly more attachment that needs to be lost prior to extraction being required and thus the pet has more resistance to tooth loss.

Figure 1.4 Gingivitis. The mild erythema and edema of the gingiva (marginal gingivitis) on this right maxillary fourth premolar (108) is a sure sign of gingival inflammation, and was mistakenly believed to be the first sign of disease. However, it is now known that this is a later sign, as bleeding on probing occurs before a color change (see Figure 1.5).

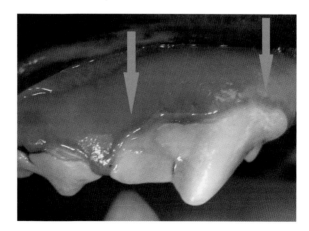

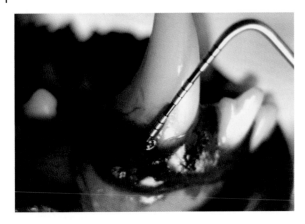

Figure 1.5 Gingivitis. This patient does not have any erythema or edema of the gingiva of this right mandibular canine (404). However, bleeding is provoked with gentle probing due to the fact that the gingiva is mildly inflamed. This is the true first sign of gingivitis, which often cannot be diagnosed without general anesthesia. Thus, gingivitis is severely underdiagnosed, which is why most veterinary dentists recommend annual cleanings regardless of conscious oral exam findings.

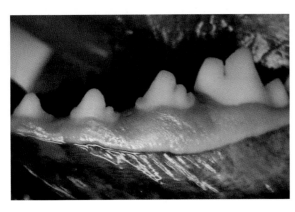

Figure 1.6 Normal gingiva. This is a picture of the mandibular left of a dog in good periodontal health. The tissues are coral pink in color and the teeth are clean.

compared to Caucasian patients [29]. Finally, several studies have identified specific genes and genomes that apparently predispose the individual to periodontal disease [30–32]. Localization of the exact genes which are responsible for specific conditions in dogs may be possible in the near future as a canine genome map is currently available [33].

1.1.2 Clinical Signs of Periodontal Disease

Normal gingival tissues are coral pink in color (allowing for normal pigmentation), and possess a smooth/regular texture (Figure 1.6). There should be no visible plaque or calculus on the dentition.

The first *clinical* sign of gingivitis is redness of the gums (see Figure 1.4), followed by edema, (Figure 1.7) and halitosis [18, 19]. However, gingival bleeding during brushing or chewing is usually noted prior to a color change, but this is hard to impossible to evaluate in a conscious patient [16, 19, 34] (see Figure 1.5). In fact, recent studies have proven that general anesthesia is required to diagnose periodontal disease, especially the earliest signs [6].

Gingivitis is typically associated with calculus, but it is caused by plaque and therefore may occur despite the absence of calculus (Figure 1.8). Alternatively, significant supragingival calculus may exist with little to no gingivitis (Figure 1.9). It is critical to understand that calculus in and of itself is essentially non-pathogenic [3, 35, 36]. Therefore, the degree of gingival inflammation should be used to judge the need for professional therapy, not the level of calculus. However, as has been previously noted, periodontal disease (especially the early stages) CANNOT be effectively diagnosed without general anesthesia [6, 9].

Figure 1.7 Gingivitis: Intraoral dental picture of the maxillary left of a canine patient with significant gingival inflammation.

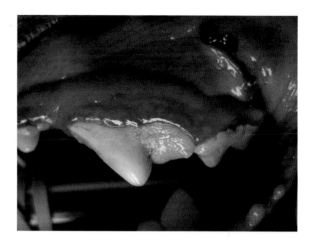

Figure 1.8 Intraoral dental picture of the maxillary right of a dog with advanced gingivitis (blue arrows) despite the fact that the teeth are fairly clean. Thus, a lack of calculus does not signify that there is no infection and the patient does not require professional intervention. This patient is in dire need of a cleaning.

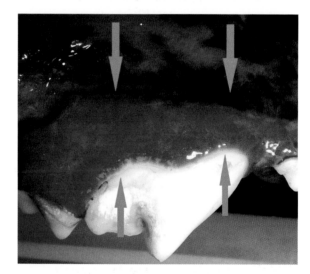

Figure 1.9 Intraoral dental picture of the maxillary right of a dog with significant calculus and minimal gingival inflammation. While this patient does require a cleaning, there is much less infection/inflammation in this case, even though there is significant dental calculus present.

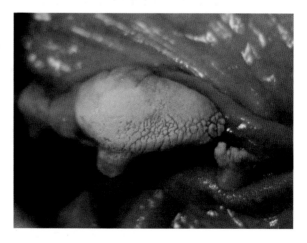

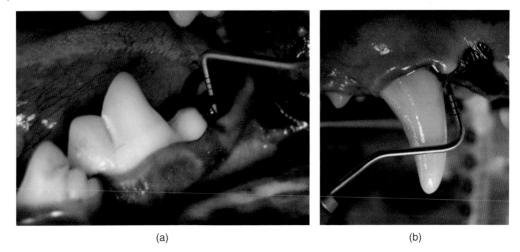

(a)   (b)

Figure 1.10 Significant attachment loss can be present in patients with clean teeth and no obvious gingival inflammation. (a) Intraoral dental picture of the mandibular left molars (309, 310) of a dog which are clean and demonstrate minimal gingival inflammation. However, periodontal probing reveals a 12-mm pocket. Both of these teeth require extraction despite appearing clean. (b) Intraoral dental picture of the right maxillary canine (104) of a dog which has minimal dental deposits and no evidence of gingivitis. However, periodontal probing reveals a 9-mm pocket. This tooth requires advanced therapy to completely resolve the infection. Ideally this consists of periodontal flap surgery and guided tissue regeneration, however extraction is an acceptable alternative.

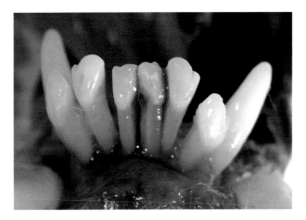

Figure 1.11 Gingival recession: Intraoral dental picture of a Yorkshire Terrier with significant gingival recession on the mandibular incisors. This may be diagnosed on conscious oral exam.

As gingivitis progresses to periodontitis (the deeper inflammation of the periodontium resulting in bone loss), the oral inflammatory changes typically intensify (however, advanced periodontal loss can be present despite normal appearing gingiva) (Figure 1.10). The hallmark feature of established periodontitis is attachment loss. There are two common presentations of attachment loss: gingival (gum) recession (Figure 1.11) and periodontal pocket formation (Figure 1.12). When recession occurs, the roots become exposed and may be identified on conscious exam. However, periodontal pockets require general anesthesia for diagnosis.

1.1.3 Onset of Periodontal Disease in Small and Toy Breed Dogs

Periodontal disease is typically thought of as a middle age to older dog problem. This is due to the fact that in most medium and large breed dogs (Cavalier King Charles Spaniels and Greyhounds

Figure 1.12 Periodontal pockets: Intraoral dental picture of the left maxillary third incisor (203) in a miniature Poodle with a deep (7-mm) periodontal pocket on the buccal aspect. Pockets virtually always require general anesthesia for accurate diagnosis.

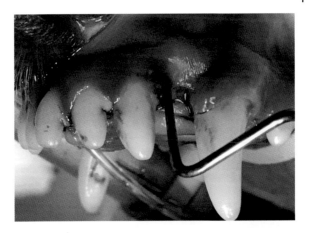

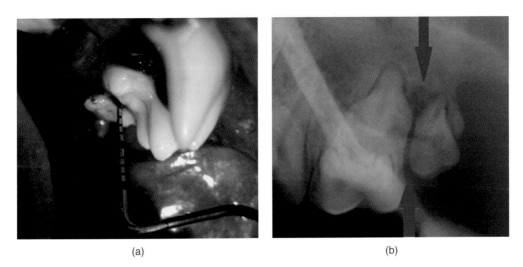

(a)   (b)

Figure 1.13 Early periodontal loss in a 3-pound poodle. (a) Intraoral dental picture of the left molars (209–10) in a 14-month-old miniature poodle. There is a 4-mm pocket present between the teeth, which in most cases would not be significant. However, the very short roots make this amount of attachment loss enough to create significant mobility and necessitate extraction of the second molar (210). (b) Intraoral dental radiograph of the area demonstrated in (a). There is significant alveolar bone loss (red arrows) between the first and second molars.

being marked exceptions (see below)), periodontal disease does not generally become significant until this time. Therefore, starting professional therapy at four to five years of age has long been an accepted practice in small animal hospitals. However, small dogs typically begin the process of periodontal bone loss very early in life [4, 5]. It has been reported that many dogs less than 10 pounds have demonstrable bone loss at just one year of age [5]. This, in combination with the decreased root length in smaller dogs, creates the need for advanced periodontal therapy (including extractions) much earlier in life. There are numerous reports of extractions being necessary in pets at one year of age (Figure 1.13). In one case treated by this author, 19 extractions were performed in a 19-month-old Pug (Figure 1.14). Furthermore, it is not unusual to perform full mouth extractions in small breed dogs prior to 4 years of age (Figure 1.15). While these are anecdotal reports, most practitioners have similar stories.

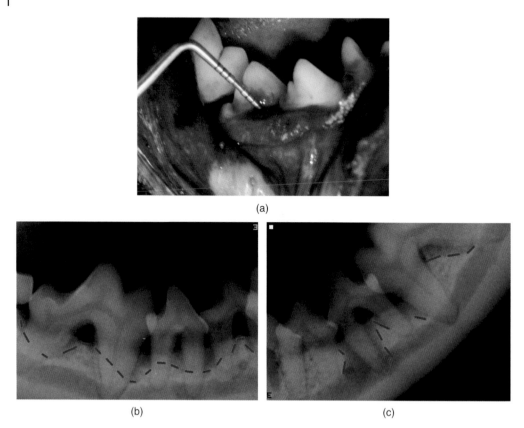

(a)

(b)   (c)

Figure 1.14 Advanced periodontal loss in an 19-month old pug. (a) Intraoral dental picture of the mandibular right premolars demonstrating significant crowding and rotation of the teeth. There is a 6-mm pocket on the fourth premolar (408), despite the fact that the teeth are fairly clean. (b and c) Intraoral dental radiograph of the right (b) and left (c) premolars/first molars of the patient. There is advanced alveolar bone loss (dashed red lines) evident on these images. Most of the imaged teeth required extraction.

1.1.4 Brachycephalic Breeds and Periodontal Disease

In general, these breeds do not appear to be more susceptible to periodontal disease than others of their size (with the exception of Cavalier King Charles Spaniels). For instance, Pugs, as small breeds, tend to suffer from periodontal disease, whereas the larger Boxers tend to be fairly resistant. However, their short maxilla typically creates crowding and rotation of the maxillary premolar teeth [37] (Figure 1.16). Crowding causes a decrease in natural cleaning ability, as well as the lack of a normal gingival collar [12]. These situations markedly increase the incidence of periodontal disease in the affected area. This is of biggest concern when the distal root of the third premolar is crowded between the mesial roots of the fourth premolar [38] (Figure 1.17). When crowding is present (especially involving the fourth premolar), extracting a tooth (the non-strategic tooth if possible) to create room will alleviate much of this issue. (For a complete discussion of rotated and crowded teeth, see below.)

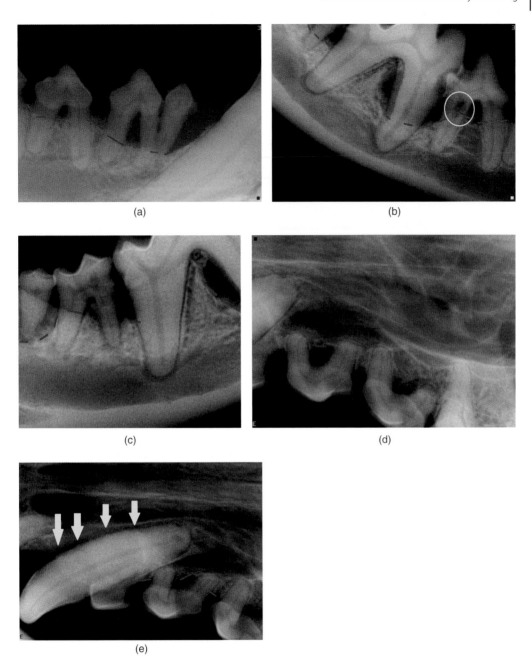

(a)

(b)

(c)

(d)

(e)

Figure 1.15 Significant periodontal bone loss in a 4-year-old miniature poodle. Dental radiographs of the mandibular right (a, b, c) and maxillary left (d & e) of the patient demonstrating significant alveolar bone loss (dashed red lines). The mandibular fourth premolar (408) already has an evident tooth resorption lesion in the distal root (yellow circle). The maxillary canine (204) has developed an oronasal fistula (yellow arrows).

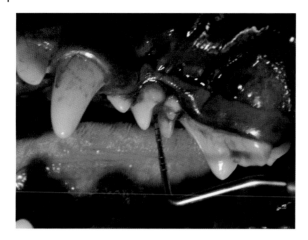

Figure 1.16 Crowing. Intraoral dental picture of a Pug with significant crowding and rotation of the left maxillary premolar teeth. This patient is less than two years old and already has gingival recession as well as a pathologic periodontal pocket.

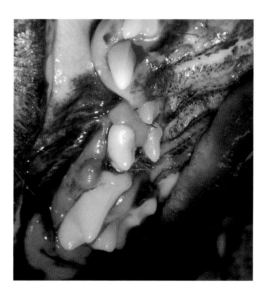

Figure 1.17 Intraoral dental picture of the right maxillary arcade in a French Bulldog with significant crowding and rotation of the maxillary premolar teeth. The distal root of the third premolar is between the mesial roots of the fourth premolar. Note the gingival recession and foreign bodies (hair) between the crowded second and third premolars.

1.1.5 Other Predisposed Breeds

Cavalier King Charles Spaniels (CKCS) and Greyhounds are well known for significant periodontal disease [26, 39]. CKCS suffer from early onset periodontal disease, especially in the maxillary premolars (as they are similar to other brachycephalic breeds). There is quite often furcation exposure of these teeth as early as two years of age. Interestingly, it is quite common for them to have advanced periodontal loss with minimal calculus and gingivitis (Figure 1.18).

Greyhounds have a different pattern of attachment loss, in that they quickly develop advanced gingival recession (Figure 1.19). This situation creates early furcational involvement as well as exposing the rougher root surfaces, both of which facilitate plaque accumulation and makes homecare more challenging. Therefore, greyhound owners must start homecare early, which is often not possible as they have often been rescued from a racetrack later in life.

Both of these breeds are very difficult to manage due to the high genetic potential for the disease. They typically suffer from significant gingivitis and early bone loss with only minimal calculus.

Figure 1.18 Intraoral dental picture of the right mandibular first molar (409) in a CKCS. The periodontal probe is demonstrating a 12-mm periodontal pocket, despite the lack of gingivitis and dental calculus. This presentation is not unusual in this breed, and therefore regular cleanings should be performed regardless of clinical signs. This tooth should be extracted to resolve the infection.

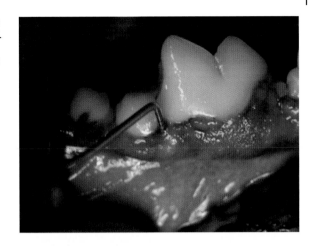

Figure 1.19 Intraoral dental picture of the right maxillary third and fourth premolars (107, 108) in a greyhound. Note that there is advanced gingival recession with minimal inflammation or dental calculus. This is a common pattern of loss in this breed, and the exposure of the cementum, which is much rougher than the enamel, leads to faster plaque accumulation and hastens the recurrence of periodontal disease following professional care. These teeth should be extracted to resolve the infection.

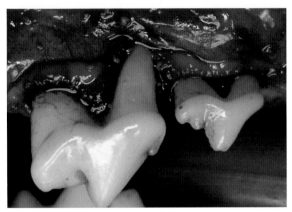

Thus, early initiation of effective and consistent homecare along with regular professional cleanings is critical to maintaining periodontal health.

1.1.6 Significant Local Ramifications of Periodontal Disease

There are several well-established local ramifications of periodontal disease [36, 40]. These include: oronasal fistulas (ONFs) [41] , class II perio-endo lesions [42, 43], pathologic mandibular fractures [18, 44], ocular problems (including eye loss) [45, 46], osteomyelitis [47, 48], and an increased risk of oral cancer [49–52]. There does not appear to be a breed predilection to the latter two, but the others are seen with much higher frequency in small breed dogs, and will be detailed below. However, the higher incidence and increased severity of periodontal disease in these breeds likely increases the frequency of neoplastic change and osteomyelitis as well.

1.1.7 Oronasal Fistulas (ONFs)

ONFs are the most common significant local consequence of periodontal disease [40, 53]. This problem is generally seen in older, small breed dogs (especially chondrodystrophic breeds such as Dachshunds and Basset Hounds), but can occur in any breed [41, 54]. ONFs are typically created by the apical progression of periodontal disease on the palatal surface of a maxillary canine [54, 55];

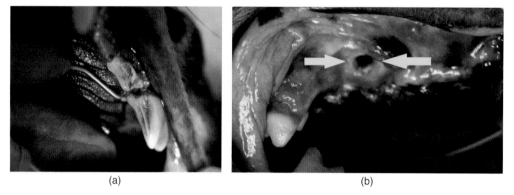

(a)   (b)

Figure 1.20 Oronasal fistulas can occur on any maxillary tooth. (The examples below actually demonstrate oroantral fistulas as the communication is caudal to the second premolar). (a) Intraoral dental picture of a fistula on the palatine surface of the left maxillary fourth premolar (208) of a Chihuahua. (b) Intraoral dental picture of a fistula from the extraction site of the right maxillary fourth premolar (108) of a miniature poodle (yellow arrows).

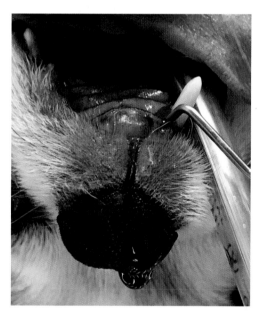

Figure 1.21   An oronasal fistula on the right maxillary canine (104) of a Chihuahua. Periodontal probing has created epistaxis from the ipsilateral nares.

(however, any maxillary tooth is a candidate) (Figure 1.20) [41]. This will eventually result in the destruction of the maxillary bone, causing a communication between the oral and nasal cavities and chronic infection (sinusitis) [40, 41, 56].

Clinical signs of an ONF include chronic nasal discharge (often hemorrhagic) (Figure 1.21), sneezing, and occasionally anorexia and halitosis [18, 41]. Occasionally, a large fistula may be noted on conscious exam (especially one that has resulted from an extraction), (Figure 1.22 and see Figure 1.20b) but definitive diagnosis of an oronasal fistula typically requires general anesthesia [41]. The diagnosis is made by introducing a periodontal probe into the periodontal space on the palatal surface of the tooth [40] (see Figure 1.21 and Figure 1.23). ONFs can occur even when the remainder of the patient's periodontal tissues are relatively healthy, including other surfaces of the affected tooth [36] (Figure 1.24 and see Figure 1.21).

Figure 1.22 Large oronasal fistula following extraction of the left maxillary canine (204) on a Dachshund (white arrows). Due to the chronic nature of the fistula, calculus has formed on the root of the third incisor (yellow arrow).

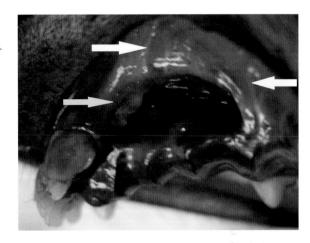

Figure 1.23 Intraoral dental picture of a periodontal probe inserted into the nasal cavity along the palatal aspect of the left maxillary canine (204) of a Basset Hound. This confirms the diagnosis of an oronasal fistula.

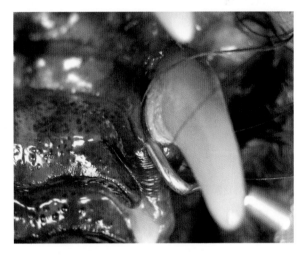

Figure 1.24 Intraoral dental picture of an oronasal fistula on the left maxillary canine (204) of a dog. There is dental calculus on the palatal aspect of the tooth, but the remainder of the tooth as well as the rest of the oral cavity is relatively healthy.

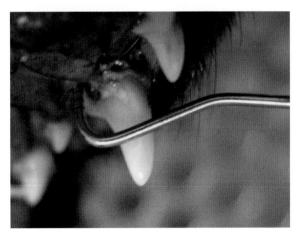

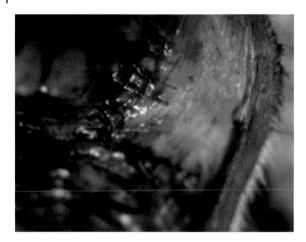

Figure 1.25 Post-operative dental picture of a single layer buccal mucosal flap created to close a chronic oronasal fistula. Lack of tension was confirmed prior to suturing.

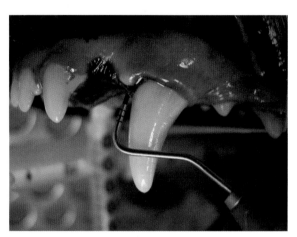

Figure 1.26 Intraoral dental picture demonstrating a 9-mm periodontal pocket on the mesio-palatine aspect of the left maxillary canine (204) in a dachshund. A fistula has not yet formed, but therapy beyond just a cleaning or closed root planning is required to remove the infection from the root surface. Periodontal flap surgery with guided tissue regeneration (preferred) or extraction is indicated.

Treatment of an ONF involves extracting the tooth (if present) and closing the defect with a *tension free* mucoperiosteal flap [41, 55, 57] (Figure 1.25). Alternatively, if a deep periodontal pocket is discovered prior to creating a communication with the nasal cavity (Figure 1.26), periodontal surgery with guided tissue regeneration may be performed to save the tooth [3, 36, 41].

1.1.8 Class II Perio-Endo Lesion

These endodontic infections are a consequence of advanced periodontal disease, and can occur in any multi-rooted tooth [18, 36, 43, 58]. They occur when the attachment loss progresses apically up the entire root, finally gaining access to the endodontic system via the apical blood supply, causing tooth death via bacterial contamination (similar to a complicated crown fracture) [18, 42, 43] (Figure 1.27). Due to the relative rarity of non-apical ramifications (blood supply other than at the apex) in veterinary patients [59], these infections do not typically occur before the infection reaches the apex. The endodontic infection subsequently spreads though the tooth via the common pulp chamber, creating periapical ramifications on the other root(s) [42, 43] However, the infected tooth may be retained by the significant surface area of the other roots(s) for an extended period of time [43].

Figure 1.27 Class II perio-endo lesion on the left mandibular second molar (310) of a dog. The periodontal loss has extended all the way to the apex of the distal root (blue arrows), allowing the oral bacteria access to the endodontic system via the previous entry point for the blood and nervous supply. This has resulted in the death of the tooth and endodontic infection which spread through the common pulp chamber and created a lesion of endodontic origin (periapical lucency) on the mesial root (red arrow).

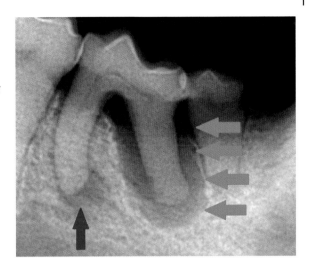

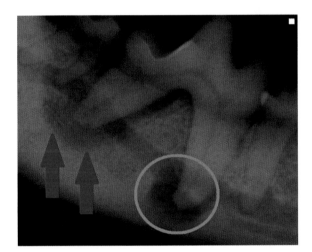

Figure 1.28 Class II perio-endo lesion on the right mandibular first molar (409) of a dog. The periodontal loss has extended all the way to the apex of the distal root (red arrows), allowing the oral bacteria access to the endodontic system via the previous entry point for the blood and nervous supply. This has resulted in the death of the tooth and endodontic infection which spread through the common pulp chamber and created a periapical lucency on the mesial root (blue circle). There is only a small amount of bone apical to the mesial root, increasing the chances of a pathologic fracture during extraction. Extreme care must be taken during the extraction attempt. Finally, note the root resorption of the distal root as well as the fact that the mesial root of the second molar is also affected.

The most common site for periodontal disease to become advanced enough without exfoliation and result in a class II perio-endo lesion is the distal root of the mandibular first molar (Figure 1.28). However, it should be noted that they can occur in any multi-rooted tooth [36, 40].

This condition is most common in older small and toy breed dogs for several reasons, most of which are detailed above [40]. First, these patients have shorter roots compared to their larger counterparts, allowing periodontal infection to reach the blood supply more readily. Second, they tend develop periodontal disease earlier. Finally, they tend to be longer living, allowing more time for bone loss to occur.

The typical treatment for class II perio-endo lesions is extraction, especially for smaller/non-strategic teeth. However, when one root of a multi-rooted tooth is significantly diseased and the other is healthy, removal of that diseased root while maintaining the healthy/healthier root/s via endodontic therapy may be desirable [42, 43].

The most common indication for root resection in veterinary dentistry is the mandibular first molar of small and toy breed dogs [60]. There is often significant disease associated with the distal root, while the mesial root is spared (Figure 1.29). There are several advantages to root resection in this presentation [61]. First, much of the crown is maintained for mastication. Second, because the distal root is often significantly diseased, its extraction is relatively atraumatic and is therefore less invasive than extracting the mesial root. Similarly, another advantage of tooth resection vs. full extraction of the mandibular first molar is the decreased risk of iatrogenic fracture [40]. With minimal bone apical to the roots in this area which has been further weakened by the periodontally induced endodontic disease, the increased force needed to extract the periodontally healthy mesial root could result in a pathologic fracture (see below).

1.1.9 Pathologic Fracture

One of the most significant local consequences of periodontal disease is a pathologic jaw fracture [18, 40, 44, 62]. These fractures typically occur in the mandible, due to chronic periodontal loss which weakens the bone in affected areas [36, 63–65] (Figure 1.30). Neoplasia and cysts (see impacted teeth below) are a possible but exceedingly rare cause of these fractures as well (Figure 1.31). These fractures can occur in any area of the mandible, but are especially common near the canines and first molars [40]. This condition is significantly more common in small breed dogs [66], owing mostly to the fact that their teeth (especially the mandibular first molar) are larger in proportion to their mandible in comparison to large breed dogs [67] (Figure 1.32). Therefore, small breed dogs have a very minimal amount of bone apical to the mandibular first molar roots (especially the mesial), putting this area at high risk of fracture when apical bone loss occurs [67].

Pathologic jaw fractures typically occur as a result of mild trauma such as falling off the couch and dog fights, however some dogs have suffered fractures while simply eating [40]. Furthermore, they often happen during dental extraction procedures (see below) [40]. This is typically considered a disease of older patients, but this author has treated several cases in dogs less than three years of age.

Pathologic fractures always carry a guarded prognosis for several reasons [40, 47, 68]. Healing is impaired by the lack of remaining bone as well as the decreased oxygen tension in the fracture site, and rigidly fixating the caudal mandible is exceedingly challenging [36, 54]. There are numerous options for fixation, but the use of wires, pins or plates is often required [40, 64]. This is because there are often no teeth caudal to the fracture for application of interdental wires or an acrylic splint. Regardless of the method of fixation, the periodontally diseased root(s) must be extracted for healing to occur [36, 47, 68] (Figure 1.33).

Awareness of the potential of pathologic fractures can aid the veterinarian during extractions in at-risk patients [40]. If one root of an affected multi-rooted tooth is periodontally healthy, there is an even greater chance of mandibular fracture due to the increased force needed to extract the healthy root [36, 43] (see Figures 1.28 and 1.29). An alternate form of treatment for these cases is to section the tooth, extract the periodontally diseased root, and perform root canal therapy on the healthy root [42, 43, 69, 70] (see Figure 1.29). In cases where severe alveolar bone loss is noted (especially if the mandibular canine or first molar is affected), it is recommended to inform the owners of

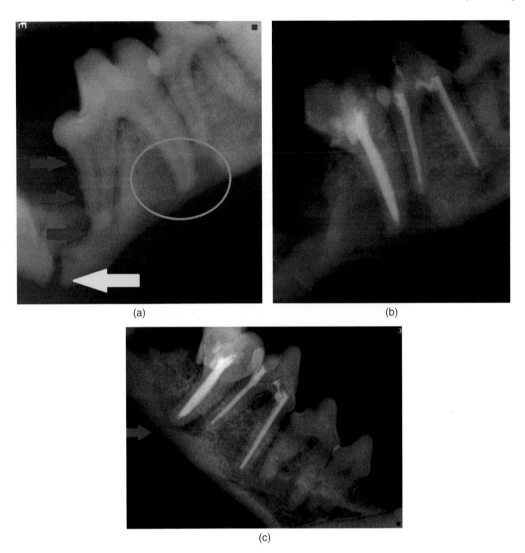

(a)

(b)

(c)

Figure 1.29 A safer option for treating severely periodontally diseased mandibular first molar.
(a) Pre-operative dental radiographs revealing extreme weakening of the mandibular bone in the apical area of the right mandibular first molar (409) in a dog. The periodontal loss has extended all the way to the apex of the distal root (red arrows), allowing the oral bacteria access to the endodontic system via the previous entry point for the blood and nervous supply. This has not only resulted in no attachment for the root, but also in the death of the tooth and endodontic infection which spread through the common pulp chamber and created a periapical lucency on the mesial root (blue circle). The bone at the apex of the mesial root is almost non-existent, and there is only a fibrous union in the area just distal to the distal root (yellow arrow). These two factors greatly increase the chances of a fracture during an extraction attempt.
(b) Post-operative dental radiograph of the patient in (a). The distal root was sectioned and easily extracted. The mesial root was treated with a root canal to avoid placing pressure on the weakened bone. Note that the fourth premolar was also non-vital and treated with root canal therapy as well. (c) 6-month recheck dental radiographs of the patient in (a & b). There is significant new bone formation in the area of the extraction, as well as almost complete resolution of the periapical lucency (red arrow). This confirmed a successful endodontic therapy and resolution of the weakened mandible.

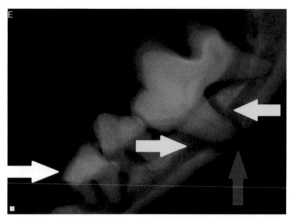

Figure 1.30   Intraoral dental radiograph of the left mandible of a 1.5 kg Yorkshire Terrier with advanced periodontal disease. This has created a complete lack of attachment on the mesial root of the first molar (309) (yellow arrows). This has resulted in a minimal amount of bone (0.3 mm) in the area (red arrow), which significantly predisposes the area to fracture (with mild trauma or during an extraction attempt). Note the complete lack of periodontal attachment of the third premolar (307) (white arrow), resulting in a "floating tooth."

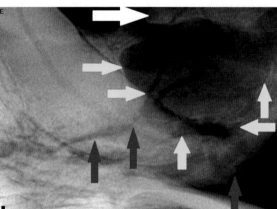

Figure 1.31   Pathologic mandibular fracture in a Boxer secondary to a dentigerous cyst. The patient had an impacted first premolar (white arrow), which has resulted in a larger dentigerous cyst (yellow arrows). The large cyst eventually weakened the jaw sufficiently to cause it to fracture (red arrows) during mild trauma (tugging on a rope).

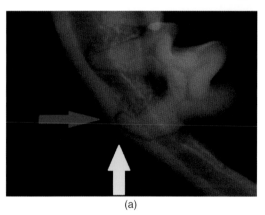
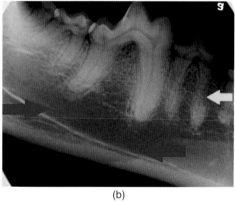

(a)   (b)

Figure 1.32   Comparison of the root anatomy of small vs. large breed dogs. (a) Normal intra-oral dental radiograph of the right mandibular first molar (409) in a 1.4 kg Maltipoo. The mesial root extends to within 0.5 mm of the ventral cortex of the mandible (yellow arrow). In addition, the root has a significant distal curve (red arrow). Both of these findings greatly increase the chances of fracture should extraction become necessary. (b) Intraoral dental radiograph of the mandibular right first molar (409) of a 37 kg German Shepherd Dog. There is significant (2.5 cm) of bone apical to the tooth roots of the first molar (blue arrows). Thus, there would be plenty of strength left in the jaw even if the periodontal bone was completely lost. Mandibular fracture should not occur in these patients. Note the incidental finding of tooth resorption on the roots of the fourth premolar (408) (yellow arrow). There is no clinical evidence of the resorption, and therefore radiographic monitoring is sufficient.

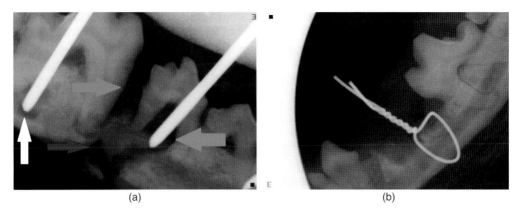

(a) (b)

Figure 1.33 Improper treatment of pathologic mandibular fractures resulted in non-union and continued infection vs, proper therapy resulting in a healed fracture site. (a) Intraoral dental radiograph of the right mandible of a Dachshund with a non-healing fracture. The patient has been repeatedly (three times) treated with an external fixator without the benefit of intraoral dental radiographs. This has resulted in failure of fixation and non-union (red arrow). The dental radiographs revealed that there was advanced periodontal disease affecting the fourth premolar and first molar (408 & 409), which was not allowing the bone to heal. Finally, there was damage to and infection of the teeth by poorly placed pins (white arrows). Removal of the appliance and extraction of the infected teeth allowed healing with minimally invasive interfragmentary wires. (b) Intraoral dental radiograph of a pathologic fracture of the mandibular left of a Miniature Poodle. The infected third and fourth premolars (307 and 308) were extracted, and then the fracture reduced and fixed with a single circum-mandibular wire.

the possibility of an iatrogenic jaw fracture prior to attempting extraction of the offending tooth [36, 40]. Referral to a veterinary dentist for extraction of these teeth is strongly encouraged.

1.1.10 Ocular Damage

Another local ramification of advanced periodontal disease results from inflammation close to the orbit which can potentially lead to ocular inflammation, nasolacrimal disease, retrobulbar abscesses, and potentially blindness [36, 40, 45, 46] (Figure 1.34). The proximity of the tooth root

Figure 1.34 Chronic right eye infection in a 5 kg mixed breed brachycephalic dog.

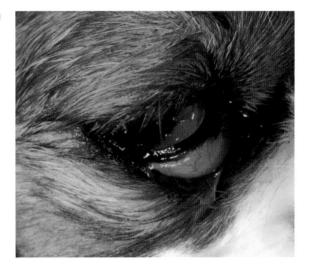

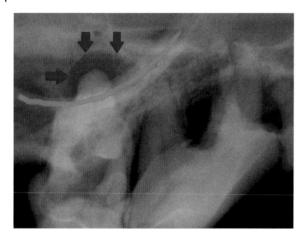

Figure 1.35 Intraoral dental radiograph of the right maxillary first molar (109) in the patient in Figure 1.34. The globe is outlined by the green line. The tooth has a large periapical lucency affecting the palatal root, which resides very close to the globe. The chronic infection almost resulted in enucleation, but was resolved with extraction of the tooth.

apices of the maxillary molars and fourth premolars to the orbit places the delicate optic tissues in jeopardy [46, 71], (Figure 1.35).

1.1.11   Systemic Consequences of Periodontal Disease [72]

While no current research supports that systemic effects of periodontal disease are increased in small and toy breed dogs, there are two facts that may lead to intensification of systemic effects in these breeds. First, as discussed, they typically suffer from a more significant level of disease. Secondly, their larger proportional periodontal surface area provides increased systemic spread compared to body size of larger breeds or human beings.

Systemic ramifications of periodontal disease have been extensively studied over the last few decades, which has resulted in a plethora of publications in peer-reviewed journals. While most of the research has been performed on humans, there is an increasing number of veterinary papers. In addition, while there is currently no proof of cause and effect, there is mounting evidence of the negative consequences of periodontal disease on the systemic health of human and animal patients.

The pathogenesis of the systemic affects is based on the inflammatory cascade. In response to the bacterial infection, the patient creates inflammation within the gingival/periodontal tissues to allow the body's defenses to attack the subgingival bacteria. However, this inflammation not only further inflames the periodontal tissues, it also allows bacteria to gain ready access to the bloodstream and thus to the entire body [73–75]. This is due to enlarged space between the crevicular epithelial cells and increased vascular permeability.

Not only do the bacteria cross the gingival barrier, but also the inflammatory mediators they produce, such as lipopolysaccharides (LPS). The bacteria and their noxious byproducts can create significant deleterious effects throughout the entire body [76]. In addition to the bacteria themselves and their toxic byproducts, systemic effects are also driven by the patient's activation of its own inflammatory mediators such as cytokines (TNF, PGE2, IL-1, and 6) [77–79]. The effect of these pro-inflammatories on the systemic health of the patient is demonstrated by numerous studies on inflammatory markers in periodontal disease and their response to therapy in both human and veterinary patients [77, 80–82].

Periodontal disease has been linked to numerous systemic problems such as cardiovascular (Figure 1.36), hepatic (Figure 1.37), and renal (Figure 1.38) dysfunction and disease in both veterinary and human studies [7, 77, 80, 83–90]. In addition, human research has revealed associations

Figure 1.36 Post-mortem picture of valvular endocarditis in a miniature Poodle. The patient died of congestive heart failure and had significant periodontal disease. Source: Photo courtesy of Dr. Joao Orvahlo and was previously published in "Veterinary Dental Applications in Emergency Medicine and Critical or Compromised Patients." Used with permission from Practical Veterinary Publishing.

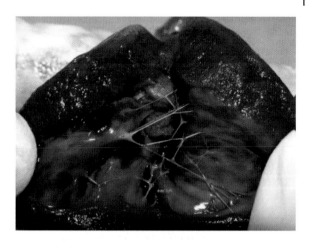

Figure 1.37 Post-mortem picture of areas of abscessation on the liver of a canine patient with multiple organ failure. Source: Images courtesy of Dr. Jerzy Gawor and was previously published in "Veterinary Dental Applications in Emergency Medicine and Critical or Compromised Patients." Used with permission from Practical Veterinary Publishing.

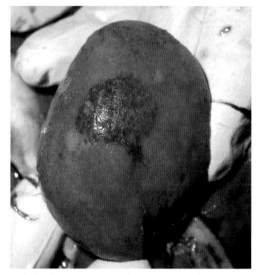

with cardiac disease, strokes, arthritis, diabetes, pulmonary disease, adverse pregnancy affects, and anemia of chronic disease [75, 91–104].

Recent studies also propose a link between periodontal disease and distant neoplasia such as gastrointestinal, kidney, pancreatic, and hematological cancers [105–109]. Further papers show that human patients affected with periodontal disease are four times more likely to have multiple (three or more) systemic issues than those with good periodontal health [110]. A striking indicator of the degree that periodontal disease negatively affects overall health is established in mortality studies. In several peer-reviewed studies, periodontal disease has been shown to be a significant predictor of hastened mortality in humans [111–113]. One study from Scandinavia reported that severe periodontal disease is actually a higher risk factor for early death than smoking [114].

1.1.12 Systemic Benefits of Periodontal Therapy

It is quite common for canine pet parents whose dogs develop comorbidities (systemic health issues) to express their desire to avoid anesthesia. In addition, many veterinarians are reluctant to anesthetize these patients. These pervasive fears emanate from the myths that anesthesia carries

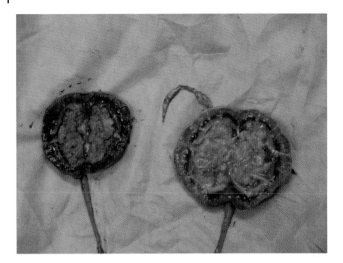

Figure 1.38 Gross necropsy picture of kidneys with severe glomerulonephritis from a patient who died of renal failure. The patient also had severe periodontal disease which may have contributed to the systemic infection and organ dysfunction. Previously published in "Veterinary Dental Applications in Emergency Medicine and Critical or Compromised Patients." Source: Used with permission from Practical Veterinary Publishing.

excessive risk as comorbidities develop, or that morbidity and/or mortality increases significantly with age. Further, there has been no perception of significant benefit of dental care and thus those perceived risks are not balanced by the potential benefits derived from proper dental care.

However, it has been shown that age in and of itself has minimal effect on anesthetic morbidity and mortality, other than being clearly associated with comorbidities which do increase anesthetic risk [115, 116]. Further, most comorbidities (even heart disease) carry minimal additional anesthetic risk and the vast majority of pets can still undergo anesthesia, provided it is properly performed and monitored [117]. Finally, recent studies have proven that treating periodontal disease in these patients will improve their overall health (see below).

By far the best studied conditions are diabetes and heart disease in humans. Proper therapy of periodontal disease has been shown to improve glycemic control as well as decrease insulin requirements [118–120]. Conversely, periodontal health is improved in patients with good diabetic control [121, 122]. There is also evidence to suggest that periodontal therapy improves renal function [123, 124]. Furthermore, periodontal therapy has been shown to improve liver values and increase lifespan in patients with cirrhosis [118, 125–127]. Periodontal therapy also has been shown to decrease the level of circulating inflammatory products and improve endothelial function in people [128, 129]. Further studies in the veterinary literature indicate that systemic inflammatory markers and oxidative stress were decreased following periodontal therapy [80, 130].

These studies demonstrate the value of periodontal care in patients with comorbidities as well as the minimal anesthetic risk associated with them. Therefore, clients should be *encouraged* to pursue therapy in all but cases of severe systemic disease. If the practitioner is concerned about the anesthesia risk, referral to a veterinary dentist is recommended. This is because they can typically perform the procedure faster, often practice within a large referral clinic, and may have access to an anesthesiologist. For a list of Board-Certified Veterinary Dentists visit www.AVDC.org.

Conclusions

Periodontal disease is almost ubiquitous in small and toy breed dogs, starting well before one year of age. In addition, the shorter roots often make extractions necessary very early in life. The small, fragile jaws result in numerous significant local ramifications such as oronasal fistulas and pathologic fractures, which are almost unheard of in larger dogs. These situations, in combination with the severe systemic effects represent a significant animal welfare concern (see Chapter 3). Therefore, early and regular intervention is mandated for the long-term health of these patients. For information on therapy of periodontal disease in small and toy breed dogs, please see Chapter 10.

Editor's note: This was a brief synopsis of periodontal disease and mostly specific to small breed dogs. Practitioners should not rely on this text as sufficient for a complete understanding of periodontal disease. For more information on this disease process and its treatment the reader is directed to the Wiley text "Veterinary Periodontology" by Dr. Brook A. Niemiec.

1.2   Persistent Deciduous (PD) Teeth

A deciduous tooth is considered persistent as soon as the permanent tooth begins to erupt into the mouth [131]. This means that the permanent tooth does not need to be fully erupted for the deciduous to be considered persistent [132, 133]. This condition is far more common in toy and small breed dogs, and Yorkshire Terriers appear particularly predisposed [131, 134]. This is likely due to the change in the facial structures created by specialized line breeding [135].

The most common cause for a deciduous tooth to be persistent is an incorrect eruption path of the permanent tooth [131, 135]. When the permanent tooth erupts along its natural path, it places pressure on the apex of the deciduous tooth resulting in apical resorption in the deciduous tooth [48, 136]. The steady coronal advancement of the permanent tooth will result in continued resorption of the deciduous. This progresses until the deciduous root is sufficiently resorbed, at which point it exfoliates, and the permanent tooth assumes its normal position in the mouth [137].

When a permanent tooth follows an unnatural path, there will be no impetus for the root of the deciduous tooth to resorb [138]. This results in the deciduous tooth remaining in the arcade with the permanent tooth erupting alongside. This improper path is currently considered to be genetic because of the pattern of occurrence within specific breeds and skull types [135].

Persistent deciduous dentition is typically bilateral. The most common teeth to be persistent are the canines, the incisors are next most common, and finally premolars [135]. Oral exam will reveal extra teeth in the arcades, giving the appearance of crowding (Figure 1.39). In addition, the adult dentition may be in an abnormal position [131] (Figure 1.40). This unnatural position may cause tooth, gingival, or palatine trauma [131, 135]. This may also result in traumatic pulpitis in the permanent dentition [37]. Studies have shown these orthodontic problems can occur within *2 weeks* of the permanent tooth starting to erupt [132, 135].

In addition to orthodontic consequences, periodontal problems are a potential sequela of persistent deciduous teeth [16]. The most obvious reason is that the retained deciduous teeth typically create crowding. Crowding decreases the natural cleaning ability derived from chewing, thus hastening the formation of plaque and thus promoting periodontal inflammation [12, 18, 37, 139]

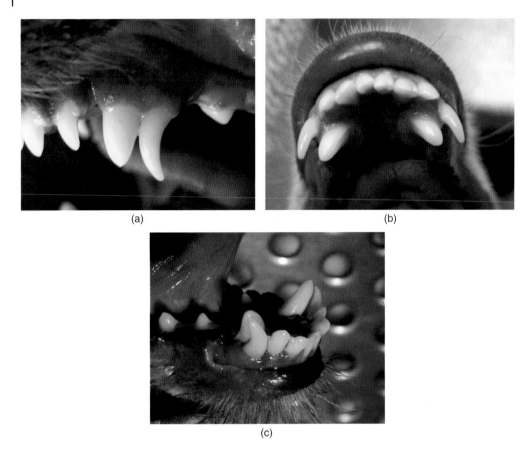

(a)

(b)

(c)

Figure 1.39 Persistent deciduous teeth. The most common appearance of persistent deciduous teeth is the appearance of an "extra" crowded tooth. Examples of a left maxillary canine (604) (a), mandibular canines (704 & 804) (b) and right mandibular canine (804) (c). Note that in a & c, there is no gingival collar between the teeth and in (b) that the permanent canines are linguocclused.

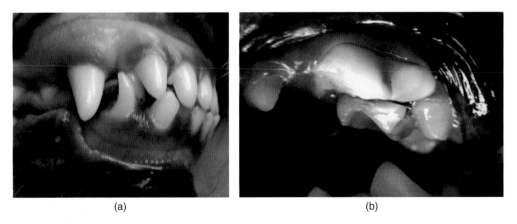

(a)

(b)

Figure 1.40 Deviation of the permanent teeth into abnormal and potentially traumatic positions by the persistent deciduous teeth. (a) The persistent deciduous right mandibular canine (804) is keeping/deflecting the permanent canine (404) lingually resulting in palatine trauma from the permanent. (b) The persistent deciduous left maxillary fourth premolar (608) is keeping/deflecting the permanent fourth premolar (208) buccally resulting in trauma to the buccal mucosa from the permanent as well as loss of normal chewing ability.

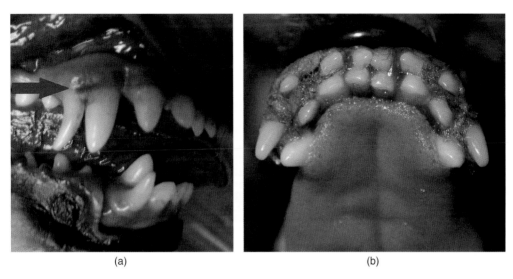

(a)   (b)

Figure 1.41   Persistent deciduous teeth hasten the onset of periodontal disease in the corresponding permanent tooth due to crowding. (a) Intraoral dental picture of a 9-month-old Yorkshire Terrier with persistent deciduous canines. The crowding has led to an early accumulation of plaque and calculus along with associated gingivitis (blue arrow). (b) Intraoral dental picture of the mandibular incisors and canines in a 12-month-old miniature Poodle. All 6 deciduous incisors and both canines are persistent. The crowding has resulted in significant accumulation of foreign bodies (hair) as well as significant inflammation and infection.

Figure 1.42   Persistent teeth do not allow for normal maturation of the gingiva, resulting in early periodontal attachment loss. This is an intraoral dental picture of the right mandibular canines (804 and 404) in a 16-month-old Yorkshire Terrier. The crowding has resulted in a rapid loss of periodontal attachment, creating a 9-mm pocket in a very young dog. Advanced therapy (periodontal flap surgery and guided tissue regeneration) was required along with extraction of the deciduous tooth. Alternatively, the permanent canine could also have been extracted.

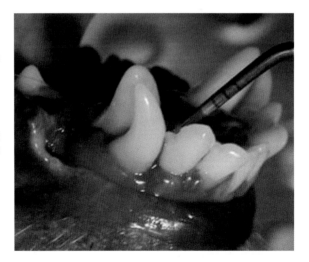

(Figure 1.41). A hidden, but perhaps even more important situation comes from the fact that the deciduous and permanent teeth share the same gingival collar [132]. The lack of a maturation of the gingiva with the permanent tooth results in a weakened periodontal attachment and thus increased susceptibility to periodontal disease [131, 135] (Figure 1.42). Human studies report that this periodontal damage starts *within 48 hours* of the permeant tooth *starting* to erupt [131, 132]. These findings mean that retained deciduous teeth in small and toy breed dogs are even more concerning because as previously discussed, these patients are also more prone to periodontal disease.

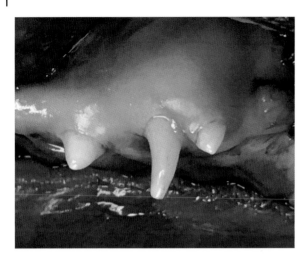

Figure 1.43 The permenent tooth does not need to be fully erupted for the deciduous to be considered persistent. As soon as any part of the permanent tooth is visible, it is considered persistent and extraction is indicated.

These significant ramifications make prompt therapy of PD teeth a medical priority. Remember, the permanent tooth does not need to be completely erupted for these problems to occur [132]. In fact, problems begin as soon as the permanent tooth starts to erupt (Figure 1.43). Therefore, timely extraction of these teeth is of vital importance, especially in small and toy breeds. *There should never be two teeth of the same type in the same place at the same time* [132].

In the past, these teeth would be dealt with at the time of neutering. However, given that the canine teeth erupt at four to five months of age and neutering rarely occurs prior to six months of age, the delay can create significant damage. Furthermore, there is a trend towards delaying or completely avoiding neutering, thus making this no longer an acceptable practice.

1.2.1 Treatment

PD teeth should be extracted as expediently as possible to help avoid the periodontal and orthodontic ramifications [140]. For small and toy breed dogs, it is recommended to have the clients monitor the maxillary canines for eruption. As soon as the permanent canines begin erupting, the pet should be presented to a veterinarian for evaluation and extraction if necessary.

Extractions of deciduous teeth can be very difficult as the roots are proportionally much longer and thinner than in the corresponding permanent dentition [141, 142] (Figure 1.44). Deciduous extractions must be performed very carefully and gently with a large amount of patience [141, 143, 144].

Another reason to be cautious during deciduous extractions is to avoid damaging the developing permanent tooth [140, 141]. Prior to eruption, the immature enamel is very susceptible to damage which can easily be caused by an elevator, and once damaged cannot be naturally repaired [145–147]. This can result in enamel hypocalcification, which exposes the dentin and leads to pain and possible infection (Figure 1.45a) [148–152]. In addition, the roughened tooth surface can hasten the accumulation of plaque and calculus and thus speed the development of periodontal disease [18, 146, 153]. If this occurs, the affected teeth should be restored, either with a bonded sealant or composite restoration (Figure 1.45b).

Dental radiographs are absolutely critical to extracting deciduous teeth [138, 154]. Deciduous teeth will often undergo some to significant resorption, typically due to the pressure placed on it

Figure 1.44 Deciduous teeth are much longer and thinner than permanent teeth. This image demonstrates the relative size of the crown (left of the red line) and root (right of the red line) on a deciduous maxillary canine (top) and first incisor (bottom). Client education as to the size of these roots is important for increasing compliance.

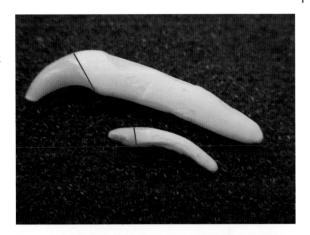

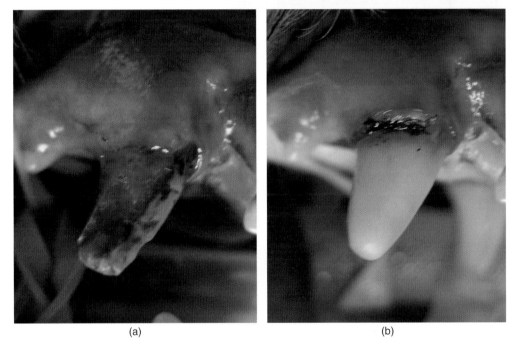

(a)   (b)

Figure 1.45 Significant damage can be caused to the permanent tooth during deciduous extractions.
(a) The permanent right maxillary canine (104) was severely damaged during extraction of the deciduous tooth. This has created not only significant sensitivity (pain) and potential endodontic infection, but in addition roughness will increase plaque and calculus attachment, hastening periodontal disease.
(b) Post-operative image of the tooth imaged in (a) following the application of a composite restoration. The restoration blocks of the pathway for pain and infection, but also smooths the tooth to retard plaque formation. Restorative dentistry is part of a comprehensive periodontal therapy protocol.

by the erupting permanent dentition (Figure 1.46). These teeth are predisposed to fracture, but an intact root canal is often still present. The resorption and potential ankylosis makes extraction very difficult, commonly resulting in a fractured root. Contrary to popular belief, intact/normal deciduous roots do NOT resorb, and will affect the patient regardless of the lack of clinical signs [132, 155] (Figure 1.47).

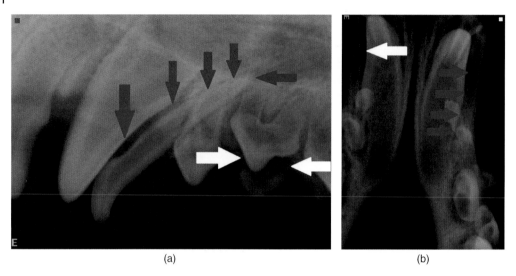

(a)   (b)

Figure 1.46 Partial resorption of persistent deciduous teeth greatly complicate extraction attempts. (a) Intraoral dental radiograph of the maxillary left of a 5-month-old dog. The permanent second premolar (206) is correctly erupting just under the deciduous causing it to be appropriately resorbed (white arrows). However, the permanent canine (204), is erupting mesial to the corresponding deciduous, thus no eruptive pressure is being applied, resulting in a normal root remaining (blue arrows). However, the lateral pressure at the gingival margin created a area of resorption at the neck of the deciduous tooth (red arrow). This cervical resorption often causes fracture of the root at the gumline. Knowledge of this situation will smooth the extraction. (b) Intraoral dental picture of the mandibular canines of a 7-month-old dog. On the right side, there is a small area of resorption at the gingival margin (white arrow), with normal roots apical to that point. The root is very weak at this point, so extreme care must be taken to avoid a root fracture. The left deciduous canine has significant resorption of the root (red arrows), but enough remaining root to require complete extraction. A surgical (open) extraction is strongly recommended from the beginning to improve the chances of successful extraction.

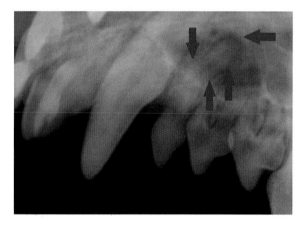

Figure 1.47 Intraoral dental radiograph of the maxillary left in a 14-year-old Maltese. This patient had been suffering from long term ocular infections. Dental radiographs revealed a retained root of the deciduous canine (604) (blue arrows). The tooth also was infected as evidenced by the periapical lucency (red arrows). Extraction of the deciduous tooth resulted in resolution of the infection. This case demonstrates the importance of complete extraction of deciduous teeth as well as dental radiography as a critical diagnostic modality for maxillofacial disease.

However, on occasion, the root of the deciduous tooth may have already been almost completely resorbed [138] (Figure 1.48). In this situation, only the crown and the very small retaining root segment need to be extracted. Having this knowledge initially, saves the practitioner time in searching for the root, avoids undue stress and worry, and avoids unnecessary surgical trauma for the patient.

Some veterinary dentists perform surgical extractions for deciduous canines to decrease the possibility of causing iatrogenic damage [131]. Most veterinary dental texts recommend closed

Figure 1.48 Intraoral dental radiograph of a persistent deciduous right mandibular canine (804). In this case, the root is completely resorbed, and the crown is only held in by the gingival attachment (red arrow). Extraction in this case is simple, and this knowledge avoids unnecessary surgical exploration for a non-existent root.

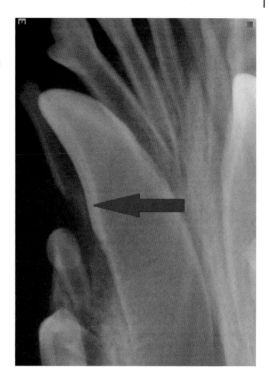

Figure 1.49 A 1.3 mm luxating elevator is a good choice for deciduous extractions.

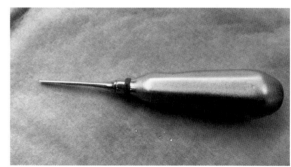

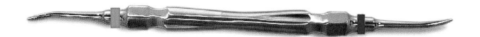

Figure 1.50 Fahrenkrug elevator is curved to correctly follow the roots of deciduous canines.

extractions in cases with significant root resorption, while a surgical approach be employed when the root appears normal [141, 148]. However, this author recommends a closed technique for the vast majority of deciduous extractions due to decreased surgical time and trauma of the surrounding tissues [141, 148]. A very small (1–2 mm) and sharp luxating elevator (Figure 1.49) used in a "rock in and twist" motion is best for these teeth [156]. Alternatively, specially designed Fahrenkrug elevators can be utilized (Figure 1.50).

Root fractures are a common complication of extractions, especially of deciduous teeth [157]. If a root breaks, every effort should be made to remove the retained piece(s) [131, 140, 148, 158]. Despite the common thought that roots of deciduous teeth resorb on their own, it is simply not true. Resorption of deciduous teeth occurs most commonly due to pressure from the erupting permanent dentition. Once the permanent crown as erupted, little to no resorption pressure will be placed on the deciduous (see above).

A retained root tip may become infected or act as a foreign body, thereby creating significant inflammation [159]. Unfortunately, there are rarely clinical signs associated with this, but retained roots are known to be painful, and often become infected [148]. Complete root tip removal is even more critical when performed for certain interceptive orthodontic purposes (especially linguoclused mandibular canines), because the apex is sufficient to deflect the permanent tooth from its normal location as well as possibly impede eruption of the permanent [148, 160]. Retained roots are best extracted utilizing a surgical (open) approach [141, 148, 156].

Post-operative dental radiographs are strongly recommended following extraction, in order to confirm complete removal of the deciduous tooth as well as the presence and proper condition of the unerupted permanent teeth [132, 157].

References

1 University of Minnesota Center for Companion Animal Health (1996). *National Companion Animal Study, Uplinks*, 3. PA, Philadelphia: Lippincott-Raven.

2 Lund, E.M., Armstrong, P.J. et al. (1999). Health status and population characteristics of dogs and cats examined at private veterinary practices in the United States. *J. Am. Vet. Med. Assoc.* 214: 1336–1341.

3 Wiggs, R.B. and Lobprise, H.B. (1997). Periodontology. In: *Veterinary Dentistry, Principals and Practice*, 186–231. Philadelphia, PA: Lippincott-Raven.

4 Fernandes, N.A., Batista Borges, A.P., Carlo Reis, E.C. et al. (2012). Prevalence of periodontal disease in dogs and owners' level of awareness - a prospective clinical trial. *Rev. Ceres. Viçosa.* 59 (4): 446–451.

5 Queck KE, Chapman A, Herzog LJ, Shell-Martin T, Burgess-Cassler A, McClure GD. (2018). Oral-Fluid Thiol-Detection Test Identifies Underlying Active Periodontal Disease Not Detected by the Visual Awake Examination. *J Am Anim Hosp Assoc.* May/Jun;54(3):132–137.

6 Wallis, C., Patel, K.V., Marshall, M. et al. (2018). A longitudinal assessment of periodontal health status in 53 Labrador retrievers. *J. Small Anim. Pract.* 59 (9): 560–569.

7 Hoffmann, T.H. and Gaengler, P. (1996). Clinical and pathomorphological investigation of spontaneously occurring periodontal disease in dogs. *J. Small Anim. Pract.* 37: 471–479.

8 Hamp, S.E., Hamp, M., Olsson, S.E. et al. (1997). Radiography of spontaneous periodontitis in dogs. *J. Periodontal Res.* 32 (7): 589–597.

9 Bauer, A.E., Stella, J., Lemmons, M., and Croney, C.C. (2018). Evaluating the validity and reliability of a visual dental scale for detection of periodontal disease (PD) in non-anesthetized dogs (*Canis familiaris*). *PLoS One* 13 (9): e0203930.

10 O'Neill, D.G., Ballantyne, Z.F., Hendricks, A. et al. (2019). West Highland white terriers under primary veterinary care in the UK in 2016: demography, mortality and disorders. *Canine. Genet. Epidemiol.* 6: 7.

11 Wallis, C., Pesci, I., Colyer, A. et al. A longitudinal assessment of periodontal disease in Yorkshire terriers. *BMC Vet. Res.* 15 (1): 207.

12 Wetering, A.V. (2011). Dental and oral cavity. In: *Small Animal Pediatrics* (eds. M.E. Peterson and M.A. Kutzler), 340–348. St. Louis, MO: Elsevier.

13 O'Neill, D.G., Church, D.B., PD, M.G. et al. (2013). Longevity and mortality of owned dogs in England. *Vet. J.* 198 (3): 638–643.

14 Michell, A.R. (1999). Longevity of British breeds of dog and its relationships with sex, size, cardiovascular variables and disease. *Vet. Rec.* 145 (22): 625–629.

15 Bellows, J. (2004). Equipping the dental practice. In: *Small Animal Dental Equipment, Materials, and Techniques, a Primer*, 13–55. Blackwell.

16 Niemiec, B.A. (2012). Etiology and pathogenesis of periodontal disease. In: *Veterinary Periodontology* (ed. B.A. Niemiec), 18–34. Ames: Wiley.

17 Fiorellini, J.P., Ishikawa, S.O., and Kim, D.M. (2006). Clinical features of gingivitis. In: *Carranza's Clinical Periodontology*, 362–372. St. Louis, MO: WB Saunders.

18 Debowes, L.J. (2010). Problems with the gingiva. In: *Small Animal Dental, Oral and Maxillofacial Disease, a Color Handbook* (ed. B.A. Niemiec), 159–181. London, Manson.

19 Fiorellini, J.P., Ishikawa, S.O., and Kim, D.M. (2006). Gingival Inflammation. In: *Carranza's Clinical Periodontology*, 355–361. St. Louis, MO: WB Saunders.

20 Meitner, S.W., Zander, H., Iker, H.P. et al. (1979). Identification of inflamed gingival surfaces. *J. Clin. Periodontol.* 6: 93.

21 Cozzi, B., Ballarin, C., Mantovani, R., and Rota, A. (2017). Aging and veterinary Care of Cats, dogs, and horses through the Records of Three University Veterinary Hospitals. *Front. Vet. Sci.* 4: 14.

22 Bonnett, B.N. and Egenvall, A. (2010 Jan). Age patterns of disease and death in insured Swedish dogs, cats and horses. *J. Comp. Pathol.* 142 (Suppl 1): S33–S38.

23 Struillou, X., Boutigny, H., Soueidan, A., and Layrolle, P. (2010). Experimental animal models in periodontology: a review. *Open. Dent. J.* 4: 37–47.

24 Marshall, M.D., Wallis, C.V., Milella, L. et al. (2014). A longitudinal assessment of periodontal disease in 52 miniature schnauzers. *BMC Vet. Res.* 10: 166.

25 O'Neill, D.G., Butcher, C., Church, D.B. et al. (2019). Miniature schnauzers under primary veterinary care in the UK in 2013: demography, mortality and disorders. *Canine Genet. Epidemiol.* 6: 1.

26 O'Neill, D.G., Rooney, N.J., Brock, C. et al. (2019). Greyhounds under general veterinary care in the UK during 2016: demography and common disorders. *Canine. Genet. Epidemiol.* 6: 4.

27 Michalowicz, B.S., Aeppli, D., Virag, J.G. et al. (1991). Periodontal findings in adult twins. *J. Periodontol.* 62 (5): 293–299.

28 Michalowicz, B.S., Aeppli, D.P., Kuba, R.K. et al. (1991). A twin study of genetic variation in proportional radiographic alveolar bone height. *J. Dent. Res.* 70 (11): 1431–1435.

29 Löe, H. and Brown, L.J. (1991). Early onset periodontitis in the United States of America. *J. Periodontol.* 62 (10): 608–616.

30 Chatzopoulos, G., Doufexi, A.E., Wolff, L., and Kouvatsi, A. (2018). Interleukin-6 and interleukin-10 gene polymorphisms and the risk of further periodontal disease progression. *Braz. Oral Res.* 32: e11.

31 Aarabi, G., Zeller, T., Seedorf, H. et al. (2017). Genetic susceptibility contributing to periodontal and cardiovascular disease. *J. Dent. Res.* 96 (6): 610–617.

32 Munz, M., Chen, H., Jockel-Schneider, Y. et al. (2017). A haplotype block downstream of plasminogen is associated with chronic and aggressive periodontitis. *J. Clin. Periodontol.* 44 (10): 962–970.

33 Mellersh, C. (2008). Give a dog a genome. *Ve.t J.* 178 (1): 46–52. Epub 2007 Sep 11.

34 Meitner, S.W., Zander, H., Iker, H.P. et al. (1979). Identification of inflamed gingival surfaces. *J. Clin. Period.* 6: 93–97.

35 Niemiec, B.A. (2013). Pathogenesis and Etiology of periodontal disease. In: *Veterinary Periodontology* (ed. B.A. Niemiec), 18–34. Ames: Wiley Blackwell.

36 Niemiec, B.A. (2008). Periodontal disease. *Top. in Comp. Ani. Med.* 23 (2): 72–80.

37 Hale, F.A. (2005). Juvenile veterinary dentistry. *Vet. Clin. Small Anim.* 35: 789–817.

38 Startup, S. (2013). Rotated, crowded, and Supernummery teeth. In: *Veterinary Orthodontics* (ed. B.A. Niemiec), 66–72. Tustin: Practical Veterinary Publishing.

39 Summers, J.F., O'Neill, D.G., Church, D.B. et al. (2015). Prevalence of disorders recorded in cavalier king Charles spaniels attending primary-care veterinary practices in England. *Canine Genet. Epidemiol.* 2: 4.

40 Niemiec, B.A. (2012). Local and regional consequences of periodontal disease. In: *Veterinary Periodontology* (ed. B.A. Niemiec), 69–80. Ames: Wiley.

41 Niemiec, B.A. (2010). Pathologies of the oral mucosa. In: *Small Animal Dental, Oral, and Maxillofacial Disease, a Color Handbook* (ed. B.A. Niemiec), 183–198. London: Manson.

42 Wang, H.L. and Glickman, G.N. (2002). *Endodontic and Periodontic Interrelationships, in Pathways of the Pulp*, 651–664. St. Louis, MO: Mosby.

43 DuPont, G.G. (2010). Problems with the dental hard tissues. In: *Small Animal Dental, Oral and Maxillofacial Disease, a Color Handbook* (ed. B.A. Niemiec), 127–157. London: Manson.

44 Mulligan, T.W., Aller, S., and Williams, C.E. (1998). *Trauma, in Atlas of Canine and Feline Dental Radiography*, 176–183. Trenton, NJ: Veterinary Learning Systems.

45 Anthony, J.M.G., Sammeyer, L.S., and Laycock, A.R. (2010). *Vet. Opthamol.* 13: 106–109.

46 Ramsey, D.T., Marretta, S.M., Hamor, R.E. et al. (1996). Ophthalmic manifestations and complications of dental disease in dogs and cats. *J. Am. Anim. Hosp. Assoc.* 32 (3): 215–224.

47 Taney, K.G. and Smith, M.M. (2010). Problems with muscles, bones, and joints. In: *Small Animal Dental, Oral, and Maxillofacial Disease, a Color Handbook* (ed. B.A. Niemiec), 199–204. London: Manson.

48 Wiggs, R.B. and Lobprise, H.B. (1997). *Veterinary Dentistry, Principals and Practice*, 128–163. Philadelphia, PA: Lippincott-Raven.

49 Rosenquist, K. (2005). Risk factors in oral and oropharengeal squamous cell carcinoma: a population-based case-control study in southern Sweden. *Swed. Dent. J. Suppl.* 179: 1–66.

50 Rosenquist, K., Wennerberg, J., Schildt, E.B. et al. (2005). Oral status, oral infectionsand some lifestyle factors for oral and oropharengeal squamous cell carcinoma. A population-based case-controlled study in southern Sweden. *Acta Otolaryngol.* 125 (12): 1327–1336.

51 Zheng, T.Z., Boyle, P., Hu, H.F. et al. (1990). Dentition, oral hygiene, and risk of oral cancer: a case-control study in Beijing, People's Republic of China. *Cancer Causes Con.* 1: 235–241.

52 Graham, S., Dayal, H., Rohrer, T. et al. (1977). Dentition, diet, tobacco, and alcohol in the epidemiology of oral cancer. *J. Natl. Cancer Inst.* 59: 1611–1618.

53 Soukup, J.W., Snyder, C.J., and Gengler, W.R. (2009). Free auricular cartilage autograft for repair of an oronasal fistula in a dog. *J. Vet. Dent.* 26 (2): 86–95.

54 Holmstrolm, S.E., Frost, P., and Eisner, E.R. (1998). Exodontics. In: *Veterinary Dental Techniques*, 2e, 215–254. Philadelphia, PA: Saunders.

55 Marretta, S.M. and Smith, M.M. (2005). Single mucoperiosteal flap for oronasal fistula repair. *J. Vet. Dent.* 22 (3): 200–205.

56 Stepaniuk, K.S. and Gingerich, W. (2015). Suspect Odontogenic infection Etiology for canine Lymphoplasmacytic rhinitis. *J. Vet. Dent.* 32 (1): 22–29.

57 Smith, M.M. (2000). Oronasal fistula repair. *Clin.Tech. Small Anim. Pract.* 15 (4): 243–250.

58 Wiggs, R.B. and Lobprise, H.B. (1997). Basic endodontic therapy. In: *Veterinary Dentistry, Principals and Practice*, 280–324. Philadelphia, PA: Lippincott-Raven.

59 Gioso, M.A., Knobl, T., Venturini, M.A., and Correa, H.L. (1997). Non-apical root canal ramifications in the teeth of dogs. *J. Vet. Dent.* 14 (3): 89–90.

60 Niemiec, B.A. (2001). Treatment of mandibular first molar teeth with endodontic-periodontal lesions in a dog. *J. Vet. Dent.* 18 (1): 21–25.

61 Theuns, P. (2012). Furcation involvement and treatment. In: *Veterinary Periodontology* (ed. B.A. Niemiec), 289–296. Ames: Wiley.

62 Startup, S. Wire-composite splint for luxation of the maxillary canine tooth. *J. Vet. Dent.* 27: 198–202.

63 Marretta, S.M. (1987). The common and uncommon clinical presentations and treatment of periodontal disease in the dog and cat. *Semin. Vet. Med. Surg. (Small Anim)* 2 (4): 230–240.

64 Snyder, C.J., Bleedorn, J.A., and Soukup, J.W. (2016). Successful treatment of mandibular nonunion with cortical allograft, Cancellous autograft, and locking titanium Miniplates in a dog. *J. Vet. Dent.* 33 (3): 160–169.

65 Bellows, J. (2004). Oral surgical equipment, materials, and techniques. In: *Small Animal Dental Equipment, Materials, and Techniques, a Primer*, 297–361. Blackwell.

66 Mulligan, T., Aller, S., and Williams, C. (1998). *Atlas of Canine and Feline Dental Radiography*, 176–183. Trenton, New Jersey: Veterinary Learning Systems.

67 Gioso, M.A., Shofer, F., Barros, P.S., and Harvery, C.E. Mandible and mandibular first molar tooth measurements in dogs: relationship of radiographic height to body weight. *J. Vet. Dent.* 18 (2): 65–68.

68 Marretta, S.M. (2012). Maxillofacial fracture complications. In: *Oral and Maxillofacial Surgery in Dogs and Cats* (eds. V. FJM and M. Lommner), 333–342. Philadelphia: Elsevier.

69 Wiggs, R.B. and Lobprise, H.B. (1997). Advanced endodontic therapy. In: *Veterinary Dentistry, Principals and Practice*, 325–350. Philadelphia, PA: Lippincott-Raven.

70 Niemiec, B.A. (2001). Treatment of mandibular first molar teeth with endodontic-periodontal lesions in a dog. *J. Vet. Dent.* 18 (1): 21–26.

71 Smith, M.M. et al. (2003). Orbital penetration associated with tooth extraction. *J. Vet. Dent.* 20 (1): 8–17.

72 Niemiec, B.A. (2012). Systemic Manafestations of periodontal disease. In: *Veterinary Periodontology* (ed. B.A. Niemiec), 81–90. Ames, IA: Wiley.

73 Scannapieco, F.A. (2004). Periodontal inflammation: from gingivitis to systemic disease? *Compend. Contin. Educ. Dent.* 25 (1): 16–25.

74 Mealy, B.L. (1999). Influence of periodontal infections of systemic health. *Periodontology* 21: 197.

75 Mealey, B.L. and Klokkevold, P.R. (2006, 2006). Periodontal medicine: impact of periodontal infection on systemic health. In: *Carranza's Clinical Periodontology*, 312–329. St. Louis, MO: WB Saunders.

76 Takai, T. (2005). Fc receptors and their role in immune regulation and autoimmunity. *J. Clin. Immunol.* 25: 1–18.

77 Pavlica, Z., Petelin, M., Juntes, P. et al. (2008). Periodontal disease burden and pathological changes in the organs of dogs. *J. Vet. Dentistry.* 25 (2): 97–108.

78 Rawlinson, J.E., Reiter, A.M., and Harvey, C.E. (2005). Tracking systemic parameters in dogs with periodontal disease. In: *Proceedings of the 19th Annual Veterinary Dental Forum*, 429. Orlando.

79 Lah, T.T., Babnik, J. et al. (1993). Cysteine proteinases and inhibitors in inflammation: their role in periodontal disease. *J. Period.* 64: 485–491.

80 Rawlinson, J.E., Goldstein, R.E., Reiter, A.M. et al. (2011). Association of periodontal disease with systemic health indices in dogs and the systemic response to treatment of periodontal disease. *J. Am. Vet. Med. Ass.* 238: 601–609.

81 Cotič, J., Ferran, M., Karišik, J. et al. (2017). Oral health and systemic inflammatory, cardiac and nitroxid biomarkers in hemodialysis patients. *Med. Oral. Patol. Oral. Cir. Bucal.* 22 (4): e432–e439.

82 Noack, B., Genco, R.J. et al. (2001). Periodontal infections contribute to elevated systemic C-reactive protein level. *J. Periodontol.* 72: 1221–1227.

83 Finch, N.C., Syme, H.M., and Elliott, J. (2016). Risk factors for development of chronic kidney disease in cats. *J. Vet. Inter. Med.* 30: 602–610.

84 Debowes, L.J., Mosier, D., Logan, E. et al. (1996). Association of periodontal disease and histologic lesions in multiple organs from 45 dogs. *J. Vet. Dent.* 13 (2): 57–60.

85 Taboada, J. and Meyer, D.J. (1989). Cholestasis in associated with extrahepatic bacterial infection in five dogs. *J. Vet. Intern. Med.* 3: 216–220.

86 DF, M.D., Cook, T. et al. (1986). Canine chronic renal disease: prevalence and types of glomerulonephritis in the dog. *Kidney Int.* 29: 1144–1151.

87 Glickman, L.T., Glickman, N.W., Moore, G.E. et al. (2009). Evaluation of the risk of endocarditis and other cardiovascular events on the basis of the severity of periodontal disease in dogs. *J. Am. Vet. Med. Assoc.* 234 (4): 486–494.

88 Abbott, J.A. (2008). Aquired Valvular disease. In: *Manual of Canine and Feline Cardiology (Fourth Edition)* (ed. L.P. Tilley), 110–138. St Louis, MO: Elsevier.

89 Trevejo, R.T., Lefebvre, S.L., Yang, M. et al. (2018). Survival analysis to evaluate associations between periodontal disease and the risk of development of chronic azotemic kidney disease in cats evaluated at primary care veterinary hospitals. *J. Am. Vet. Med. Ass.* 252: 710–720.

90 Pereira Dos Santos, J.D., Cunha, E., Nunes, T. et al. (2019). Relation between periodontal disease and systemic diseases in dogs. *Res Vet Sci.* 125: 136–140. https://doi.org/10.1016/j.rvsc.2019.06.007.

91 Hayes, C., Sparrow, D., Cohen, M. et al. (1998). The association between alveolar bone loss and pulmonary function: the VA dental longitudinal study. *Ann. Periodontol.* 3: 257.

92 Syrjanen, J., Peltola, J., Valtonen, V. et al. (1989). Dental infections in association with cerebral infarction in young and middle-aged men. *J. Inter. Med.* 225: 197.

93 Ekuni, D., Tomofuji, T., Irie, K. et al. (2010). Effects of periodontitis on aortic insulin resistance in an obese rat model. *Lab. Invest.* 90 (3): 348–359.

94 Benguigui, C., Bongard, V., Ruidavets, J.B. et al. (2010). Metabolic syndrome, insulin resistance, and periodontitis: a cross-sectional study in a middle-aged French population. *J. Clin. Periodontol.* 37 (7): 601–608.

95 Arbes, S.J. jr.,, Slade, G.D., and Beck, J.D. (1999). Association between extent of periodontal disease and self-reported history of heart attack: an analysis of NHANES III data. *J. Dent. Res.* 78: 1777.

96 Franek, E., Klamczynska, E., Ganowicz, E. et al. (2008). Association of chronic periodontitis with left ventricular mass and central blood pressure in treated patients with essential hypertension. *Am. J. Hypertens.* 22 (2): 203–207.

97 Geerts, S.O., Legrand, V., Charpentier, J. et al. (2004). Further evidence of the association between periodontal conditions and coronary artery disease. *J. Periodontol.* 75 (9): 1274–1280.

98 Deo, V., Bhongade, M.L., Ansari, S., and Chavan, R.S. (2009). Periodontitis as a potential risk factor for chronic obstructive pulmonary disease: a retrospective study. *Indian J. Dent. Res.* 20 (4): 466–470.

99 Scannapieco, F.A., Papandonatos, G.D., and Dunford, R.G. Associations between oral conditions and respiratory disease in a national sample survey population. *Ann. Periodontol.* 3 (1): 251–256.

100 Jeffcoat, M.K., Guers, N.C., Reddy, M.S. et al. (2002). Periodontal infection and pre-term birth: results of a prospective study. *J. Am. Dent. Assoc.* 132: 875.

101 Nibali, L., D'Aiuto, F., Griffiths, G. et al. (2007). Severe periodontitis is associated with systemic inflammation and a dysmetabolic status: a case-control study. *J. Clin. Periodontol.* 34 (11): 931–937.

102 Cheng, Z., Meade, J., Mankia, K. et al. (2017). Periodontal disease and periodontal bacteria as triggers for rheumatoid arthritis. *Best Pract. Res. Clin. Rheumatol* 31 (1): 19–30.

103 Nibali, L., Darbar, U., Rakmanee, T., and Donos, N. (2019). Anemia of inflammation associated with periodontitis: analysis of two clinical studies. *J. Periodontol.* 90: 1252–1259.

104 Naik, V., Acharya, A., Deshmukh, V.L. et al. (2010). Generalized, severe, chronic periodontitis is associated with anemia of chronic disease: a pilot study in urban, Indian males. *J. Invest. Clin. Dent.* 1 (2): 139–143.

105 Watabe, K., Nishi, M., Miyake, H., and Hirata, K. (1998). Lifestyle and gastric cancer: a case-control study. *Oncol. Rep.* 5 (5): 1191–1194.

106 Abnet, C.C., Qiao, Y.L., Mark, S.D. et al. (2001). Prospective study of tooth loss and incident esophageal and gastric cancers in China. *Cancer Causes and Control.* 12: 847–854.

107 Hujoel, P.P., Drangsholt, M., Spiekerman, C., and Weiss, N.S. (2003). An exploration of the periodontitis-cancer association. *Ann. of Epi.* 13: 312–316.

108 Michaud, D.S., Izard, J., Wilhelm-Benartzi, C.S. et al. (2013). Plasma antibodies to oral bacteria and risk of pancreatic cancer in a large European prospective cohort study. *Gut.* 62 (12): 1764–1770.

109 Maruyama, T., Tomofuji, T., Machida, T. et al. (2017). Association between periodontitis and prognosis of pancreatobiliary tract cancer: a pilot study. *Mol. Clin. Oncology.* 6 (5): 683–687.

110 Al-Emadi, A., Bissada, N., Farah, C. et al. (2006). Systemic diseases among patients with and without alveolar bone loss. *Quintessence Inter.* 37 (10): 761–765.

111 Jansson, L., Lavstedt, S., and Frithiof, L. (2002). Relationship between oral health and mortality rate. *J. Clin. Period.* 29: 1029.

112 Holm-Pedersen, P., Schultz-Larsen, K., Christiansen, N., and Avlund, K. (2008). Tooth loss and subsequent disability and mortality in old age. *J. Am. Geri. Soc.* 56 (3): 429–435.

113 Avlund, K., Schultz-Larsen, K., and Krustrup, U. (2009). Effect of inflammation in the periodontium in early old age on mortality at 21-year follow-up. *J. Am. Geri. Soc.* 57 (7): 1206–1212.

114 Garcia, R.I., Krall, E.A., and Vokonas, P.S. (1998). Periodontal disease and mortality from all causes in the VA dental longitudinal study. *Annals of Period.* 3: 339.

115 Brodbelt, D.C., Blissitt, K.J., Hammond, R.A. et al. (2008). The risk of death: the confidential enquiry into perioperative small animal fatalities. *Vet. Anaesth. Analg.* 35 (5): 365–373.

116 Brodbelt, D.C., Pfeiffer, D.U., Young, L.E., and Wood, J.L. (2008). Results of the confidential enquiry into perioperative small animal fatalities regarding risk factors for anesthetic-related death in dogs. *J. Am. Vet. Med. Assoc.* 233 (7): 1096–1104.

117 Carter, J.E., Motsinger-Reif, A.A., Krug, W.V., and Keene, B.W. (2017). The effect of heart disease on Anesthetic complications during routine dental procedures in dogs. *J. Am. Anim. Hosp. Assoc.* 53 (4): 206–213.

118 Hayashi, J., Hasegawa, A., Hayashi, K. et al. (2017). Effects of periodontal treatment on the medical status of patients with type 2 diabetes mellitus: a pilot study. *BMC Oral Health.* 21 17 (1): 77.

119 Simpson, T.C., Weldon, J.C., Worthington, H.V. et al. (2015). Treatment of periodontal disease for glycaemic control in people with diabetes mellitus. *Cochrane Database Sys. Rev.* 6 (11): CD004714.

120 Wang, T.F., Jen, I.A., Chou, C., and Lei, Y.P. (2014). Effects of periodontal therapy on metabolic control in patients with type 2 diabetes mellitus and periodontal disease: a meta-analysis. *Medicine.* 93 (28): 292.

121 Tervonen, T. and Knuuttila, M. (1986). Relation of diabetes control to periodontal pocketing and alveolar bone level. *Oral Sur. Oral Med. Oral Path.* 61: 346–349.

122 Tsai, C., Hayes, C., and Taylor, G.W. (2002). Glycemic control of type 2 diabetes and severe periodontal disease in US adult population. *Community Den. and Oral Epid.* 30: 182–192.

123 Artese, H.P., Sousa, C.O., Luiz, R.R. et al. (2010). Effect of non-surgical periodontal treatment on chronic kidney disease patients. *Braz. Oral Res.* 24 (4): 449–454.

124 Graziani, F., Cei, S., La Ferla, F. et al. (2010). Effects of non-surgical periodontal therapy on the glomerular filtration rate of the kidney: an exploratory trial. *J. Clin. Period.* 37 (7): 638–643.

125 Tomofuji, T., Ekuni, D., Sanbe, T. et al. (2009). Effects of improvement in periodontal inflammation by tooth brushing on serum lipopolysaccharide concentration and liver injury in rats. *Acta Odont. Scan. Scandinavica.* 67: 200–205.

126 Grønkjær, L.L. (2015). Periodontal disease and liver cirrhosis: a systematic review. *SAGE Open Medicine.* Sep. 9: 3.

127 Lins, L., Bittencourt, P.L., Evangelista, M.A. et al. (2011). Oral health profile of cirrhotic patients awaiting liver transplantation in the Brazilian northeast. *Transplant. Proc.* 43 (4): 1319–1321.

128 Mercanoglu, F., Oflaz, H., Oz, O. et al. (2004). Endothelial dysfunction in patients with chronic periodontitis and its improvement after initial periodontal therapy. *J. Period.* 75 (12): 1694–1700.

129 Correa, F.O., Gonçalves, D., Figueredo, C.M. et al. (2010). Effect of periodontal treatment on metabolic control, systemic inflammation and cytokines in patients with type 2 diabetes. *J. Clin. Period.* 37 (1): 53–58.

130 Akpinar, A., Toker, H., Ozdemir, H. et al. (2013 Jun). The effects of non-surgical periodontal therapy on oxidant and anti-oxidant status in smokers with chronic periodontitis. *Arch. Oral. Biol.* 58 (6): 717–723.

131 Hobson, P. (2005). Extraction of retained primary canine teeth in the dog. *J. Vet. Dent.* 22 (2): 132–137.

132 Niemiec, B.A. (2010). Pathology in the pediatric patient. In: *Small Animal Dental Oral and Maxillofacial Disease* (ed. B.A. Neimeic), 89–126. London: UK: Manson.

133 Sabri, R. (2008). Management of over-retained mandibular deciduous second molars with and without permanent successors. *World J. Orthod.* 9 (3): 209–220.

134 Gawor J. (2008). Kliniczna I radiologiczna ocena uzębienia u szczenięcia w trakcie wyrzynania. *Przypadek kliniczny. Zycie Wet.* 12.

135 Harvey, C.E. and Emily, P.P. (1993). *In: Small Animal Dentistry.* St. Louis: Mosby.

136 Wheeler, R.C. (1974). *Dental Anatomy, Physiology, and Occlusion*, 24. Philadelphia: WB Saunders.

137 Niemiec, B.A. (2008). Case based dental radiology. *Top Comp. Anim. Med.* 24 (1): 4–19.

138 Niemiec, B.A. The importance of and indications for dental radiology. In: *Practical Veterinary Dental Radiology* (eds. B.A. Niemiec, J. Gawor and V. Jekel), 5–30. CRC Press.

139 Buckley, L.A. (1972). The relationship between malocclusion and periodontal disease. *J. Periodontol.* 43 (7): 415–417.

140 Shope, B.H., Mitchell, P.Q., and Carle, D. (2019). Developmental pathology and Pedodontology. In: *Wiggs' Veterinary Dentistry Principals and Practice*, 2e (eds. H.B. Lobprise and J.R. Dodd), 63–79. Hoboken: Wiley Blackwell.

141 Wiggs, R. and Lobprise, H. (1997). Basics of orthodontics. In: *Veterinary Dentistry; Principles and Practice* (eds. R. Wiggs and H. Lobprise). Philadelphia: Lippincott-Raven.

142 Proffit, W. and Fields, H. (2000). Biological basis for endodontic therapy. In: *Contemporary Orthodontics*, 3e (eds. W. Proffit and H. Fields), 296–364. Mosby, Inc.

143 Holmstrolm, S., Fitch, P., and Eisner, E. (1998). *Restorative Dentistry in Veterinary Dental Techniques for the Small Animal Practitioner.* Saunders an Imprint of Elsevier.

144 Niemiec, B.A. (2012). *Dental Extractions Made Easier.* Tustin: Practical Veterinary Publishing.

145 Neville, B.W., Damm, D.D., Allen, C.M., and Bouquot, J.E. (2002). *In: Oral & Maxillofacial Pathology*, 2e. Philadelphia: WB Saunders.

146 Dupont, G. (2010). Pathologies of the dental hard tissues. In: *Small Animal Dental, Oral and Maxillofacial Disease-a Color Handbook* (ed. B.A. Niemiec), 128–159. London: Manson.

147 Niemiec, B.A. Indications for restorations. In: *Veterinary Restorative Dentistry for the General Practitioner* (ed. B.A. Niemiec), 36–47. San Diego, CA: Practical Veterinary Publishing.

148 Niemiec, B.A. (2013). Deciduous malocclusions. In: *Veterinary Orthodontics* (ed. B.A. Niemiec), 17–21. Tustin: Practical Veterinary Publishing.

149 Niemiec, B.A. (2010). Pathology in the Pediatric patient. In: *Small Animal Dental, Oral & Maxillofacial Disease* (ed. B.A.,. e.) Niemiec), 90–127. London: Manson Publishing Ltd.

150 Trowbridge, H.O. (1985). Intradental sensory units: physiological and clinical aspects. *J. Endo.* 11: 489–498.

151 Ceyhan, D., Kirzioglu, Z., and Emek, T. (2019). A long-term clinical study on individuals with amelogenesis imperfecta. *Niger. J. Clin. Pract.* 22 (8): 1157–1162.

152 Trowbridge, H.O., Syngcuk, K., and Hideaki, S. (2002). Structure and functions of the dentin-pulp complex. In: *Pathways of the Pulp*, 8e (eds. S. Cohen and R.C. Burns), 411–456. St Louis, MO: Mosby.

153 Perry, D.A., Schnid, M.O., and Takei, H.H. (2006). Phase I periodontal therapy. In: *Carranza's Clinical Periodontology*, 722–727. St. Louis, MO: WB Saunders.

154 Niemiec, B.A. (2011). The importance of dental radiology. *Eur. J. Comp. Anim. Pract.* 20 (3): 219–229.

155 Ulbricht, R.D., Marretta, S.M., and Klippert, L.S. (2003). Surgical extraction of a fractured, nonvital deciduous tooth in a tiger. *J. Vet. Dent.* 20 (4): 209–212.

156 Niemiec, B.A. (2013). *Dental Extractions made Easier*, 17–21. Tustin: Practical Veterinary Publishing.

157 Moore, J.I. and Niemiec, B.A. (2014). Evaluation of extraction sites for evidence of retained tooth roots and periapical pathology. *J. Am. Anim. Hosp. Ass.* 50 (2): 77–82.

158 Surgeon, T.W. (2000). Surgical exposure and orthodontic extrusion of an impacted canine tooth in a cat: a case report. *J. Vet. Dent.* 17 (2): 81–85.

159 Niemiec, B.A. (2013). *Dental Extractions Made Easier*. Tustin, CA: Practical Veterinary Publishing.

160 Fulton, A.J., Fiani, N., and Verstraete, F.J. (2014). Canine pediatric dentistry. *Vet. Clin. North Am. Small Anim. Pract.* 44 (2): 303–324.

2

Conditions Seen in Both Small and Brachycephalic Breeds; Therefore Small Brachycephalic Breeds (Pug, Lhasa Apso, Shih Tzu, etc.) Are Even More Significantly Affected

Brook A. Niemiec

Veterinary Dental Specialties and Oral Surgery, San Diego, CA, USA

2.1 Crowding and Rotation

Crowding is significantly increased in small breed dogs when compared to their larger counterparts [1, 2], as they have proportionally larger teeth in relation to their jaws in comparison to large breed dogs [3, 4] (Figure 2.1). Additionally, brachycephalic dogs often suffer from rotation malocclusion due to the shortened maxilla (Figure 2.2). This makes small breed brachycephalics particularly prone to crowding, (especially in their maxillary premolars). Crowding creates significant ramifications when the distal root of the third premolar is located between the mesial roots of the fourth premolar [2] (Figure 2.3). Furthermore, incisor crowding is quite common in small breeds (especially in the mandible) [3, 4] (see Figure 2.1). The crowding in combination with the decreased bone quality of the rostral mandible creates a quick onset of periodontal disease [5, 6].

Crowding is well-known to predispose the affected patient to periodontal disease [1, 2, 4, 6–9]. Teeth affected by rotation and crowding have lowered defenses to periodontal disease because of their propensity to trap food, plaque, and calculus. This food trap leads to local infection and inflammation [10, 11].

Periodontal disease is further promoted if the malpositioning or crowding creates infra-eruption. Infra-eruption is known to increase periodontal disease due to the creation of pseudopockets [12, 13]. Crowded teeth (especially those with infra-eruption) may have decreased amounts of attached gingiva, further predisposing the patient to periodontal disease [2]. Crowding can result in a lack of an interdental papilla, a part of the normal gingival collar between two teeth [2] (see Figure 2.2). Without this protective collar, both teeth are susceptible to periodontal disease [10]. Finally, if this condition creates direct gingival trauma, it can initiate or worsen periodontal disease [5, 14, 15].

In addition to increasing the incidence of periodontal disease, this condition can also create oral pain and damage from tooth on tooth or tooth on gum trauma [10, 12]. The chronic trauma resulting from tooth on tooth contact can lead to tooth non-vitality [2, 4]. Soft tissue defects can become infected and/or quite painful and may even result in oronasal fistulas [12, 16].

Treatment

Not all rotated and crowded teeth are problematic; many remain functional and non-painful throughout the life of the patient [12] (Figure 2.4). If the tooth or teeth are deemed problematic,

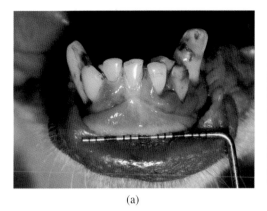

(a)

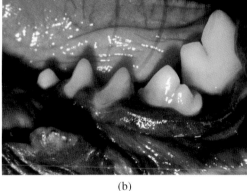

(b)

Figure 2.1 (a) Severe incisor crowding in a miniature poodle and associated periodontal disease. (b) Crowding and rotation of the left mandibular premolars of a Pug.

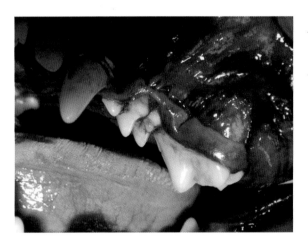

Figure 2.2 Severe crowding and rotation of the left maxillary second and third premolars (206 & 207) of an 18-month-old Pug. Note that the patient already has gingival recession due to the malocclusion.

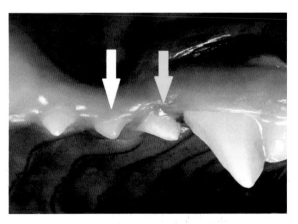

Figure 2.3 Intraoral dental picture of the maxillary left of a Pug. The third premolar (207) is erupting into the mesial furcation of the fourth premolar (yellow arrow). This crowded position will greatly hasten periodontal attachment loss of the mesial aspect of the fourth premolar. Early extraction of the third premolar will improve the long-term health of the strategic fourth premolar. Also note that the second premolar is a deciduous tooth (606) (white arrow). This tooth is likely present due to a lack of a corresponding permanent tooth (see Figure 2.6).

Figure 2.4 Intraoral dental picture of the mandibular right of a canine patient with a supernumary fourth premolar which has created rotation and crowding of the premolar teeth. Despite this fact, there is a normal gingival collar as well as spacing between all the teeth. In this situation, the teeth will likely enjoy normal natural cleaning and therefore interceptive extraction is likely not indicated.

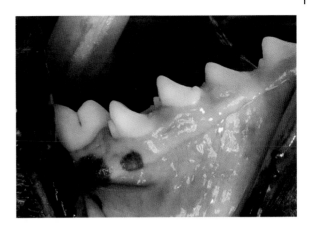

the usual treatment of choice is extraction [4]. If this is performed early in the course of the disease, the more functionally important tooth can generally be saved. For example, in the case of the rotated and/or crowded maxillary third premolar with fourth premolar (see Figure 2.1a), if the third premolar is extracted early it can save the maxillary fourth premolar [16]. Delayed treatment will often result in the extraction of both teeth due to periodontal disease.

2.2 Congenitally Missing Teeth

Hypodontia is defined as cases where several (1–5) permanent teeth are congenitally absent.

Oligodontia is when many (six or more), but not all permanent teeth do not exist from birth [17, 18]. Finally, anodontia is the congenital lack of all permanent teeth [12].

Anodontia is exceedingly rare in small animals. Hypodontia, however, is actually quite common in small and toy breeds, in particular Chinese crested, Mexican hairless, and brachycephalic breeds [18–20]. The teeth most likely to be congenitally absent in these patients are the premolars (especially 1st and 2nd), incisors, and mandibular 3rd molars [18]. The condition is also be seen in certain large breed dogs as well (especially Doberman Pinchers and German Shepherds). In dogs destined for show careers, this is considered a serious fault.

Hypodontia is considered a genetic error in tooth development [17]. However, it should be noted that developing teeth are quite susceptible to environmental forces (e.g. medications, trauma, intrauterine disturbances) [21]. Therefore developmental disturbances can also cause the lack of a tooth or several teeth in the permanent dentition. The permanent tooth develops from a bud of the deciduous tooth (except for the first premolars and all molars which do not have deciduous counterparts) [22, 23]. Consequently, if a deciduous tooth is never created, there will likewise not be a permanent tooth. However, it is more common that the deciduous tooth will have previously exfoliated. Hypodontia of the deciduous teeth is very rare.

The most common appearance of a congenitally missing tooth is an area where one or more teeth are absent [12] (Figure 2.5). However, there may be a persistent deciduous tooth in the area due to the lack of apical pressure from the erupting permanent tooth which would normally cause the deciduous root to resorb [17] (Figure 2.6).

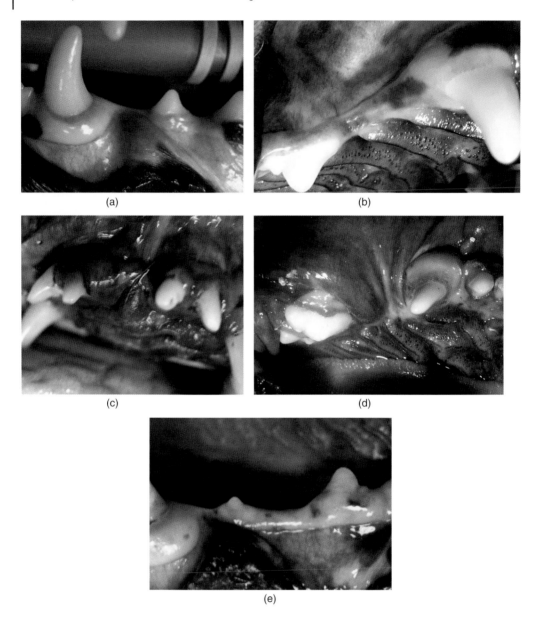

(a)   (b)

(c)   (d)

(e)

Figure 2.5 Typical appearance of "missing" teeth. Intraoral dental radiographs demonstrating a missing left mandibular first premolar (305) (a); right maxillary first and second premolars (105 & 106) (b); maxillary first incisors (101 & 201) (c); right maxillary first–third premolar (105–7) (d); and left mandibular second premolar (306) (e). Dental radiographs are required to ensure that these teeth are truly absent.

Dental radiographs are required of all "missing" teeth to confirm that they are truly absent [24] (Figure 2.7). It is critical to rule out impacted teeth, as *dentigerous cysts* may develop around unerupted teeth (see below) [21, 25] (Figure 2.8). In addition, the radiographs will identify any retained tooth roots (Figure 2.9). These are very common and often create pain and infection [26]. No treatment is required in cases of truly missing teeth.

Figure 2.6 Intraoral dental picture of the maxillary right of a dog with a deciduous second premolar (506) (blue arrow). In all likelihood, this is due to a missing permanent tooth, but radiographs should be made to confirm this. If the tooth is healthy (i.e. not undergoing resorption), it can serve as a functional tooth for a significant time or even life of the patient.

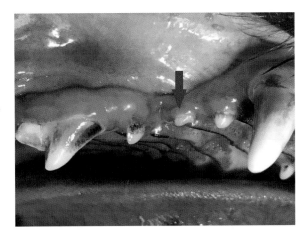

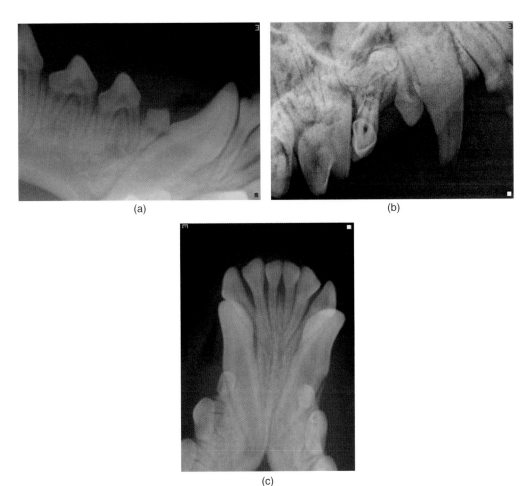

(a)

(b)

(c)

Figure 2.7 Intraoral dental radiographs of impacted teeth in dogs. Examples of the right mandibular first premolar (405) (a), right maxillary second premolar (106) (b), and mandibular canines (304, 404) (c). None of these teeth demonstrate any evidence of secondary pathology at this point.

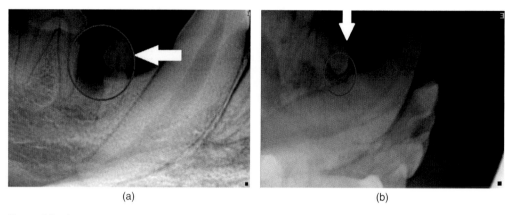

(a) (b)

Figure 2.8 Impacted teeth will commonly (29% of the time) develop dentigerous cysts. (a) & (b) Intraoral dental radiographs of impacted right mandibular first premolars (white arrows) in two dogs which reveal early dentigerous cysts (red circles). Prompt extraction of these teeth and thorough debridement of the cystic lining will avoid the expansion of these cysts and secondary complications.

2.3 Impacted or Embedded Teeth

These are teeth which do not erupt into the dentition for one of the following reasons: [12, 27]

a) Impeded by an area of thick and firm gingiva called an *operculum* (most common) [28].
b) Blocked by a structure such as bone or tooth (deciduous or permanent).
c) Failure of passive eruption.

These teeth can be malformed or normal, and are most common in brachycephalic breeds (especially small brachycephalic breeds) [12, 19, 29]. The first and second premolars are by far the most common teeth to be impacted [12, 19].

2.3.1 Treatment

If the impaction is found early (i.e. prior to apexogenesis at approximately 11–13 months of age), natural eruption is still possible [12, 30]. If the cause is soft tissue obstruction, an *operculectomy* can be performed at this time. This consists of carefully removing the soft tissue obstruction (generally with a coarse diamond bur). If the impedance is caused by teeth or bone, a more aggressive surgery of tooth/bone removal can be attempted.

If the operculectomy is unsuccessful, or the condition is not discovered until after apexogenesis is complete, it must be removed (extracted) or actively "moved." These procedures are generally more invasive than simple operculectomy. This is one of the numerous reasons for recommending that "at risk" breeds have their first dental cleaning prior to 1 year of age. While orthodontic extrusion has been described as a treatment of impacted teeth, it is a challenging procedure requiring numerous anesthesia events as well as appliance adjustments [31]. Therefore, it is rarely recommended with extraction being the treatment of choice [27]. A common question which is somewhat controversial is at what age is it "safe" to radiographically monitor impacted teeth without evidence of cystic formation. In general, if cysts are going to form, they start before three years of age. This had led to the "recommendation" of not extracting teeth in older (six years or more) patients. However, anecdotal reports of cysts developing in 10 to 12-year-old dogs exist. Further,

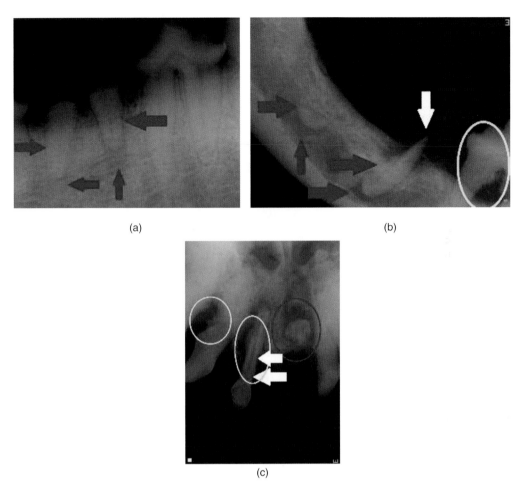

(a)   (b)

(c)

Figure 2.9 Retained tooth roots: (a) Intraoral dental radiograph of the "missing" left mandibular second premolar (306) shown in Figure 2.5e revealing retained roots (blue arrows). There is also periapical rarefaction of these roots (red arrows), indicating persistent endodontic infection. (b) Intraoral dental radiograph of a "missing" right mandibular first molar (409) revealing retained roots (blue arrows). There is also periapical rarefaction of these roots (red arrows), indicating persistent endodontic infection. The mesial root had a sharp point which was actually piercing the gingiva, creating inflammation in the area (white arrow). Finally, there is significant periodontal bone loss on the fourth premolar (408) (yellow circle) which requires extraction. (c) Intraoral dental radiograph of the "missing" maxillary first incisors (101 & 201) shown in Figure 2.5c revealing a retained root of 201 with associated bone loss (red circle), indicating persistent endodontic infection. The right second incisor (102) has a wider root canal, indicating non-vitality (white arrows). Finally, there is significant periodontal bone loss on the right second and third incisors (102 & 103) (yellow circles) which require extraction.

regular monitoring of veterinary patients is rarely performed, which significantly delays the therapy. Therefore, most veterinary dentists extract all impacted teeth. This author recommends all impacted teeth be removed in pets six years or younger. In pets over 6, if the extraction will be straightforward (i.e. the tooth is just under the soft tissue or a very thin layer of bone and will be easily located), the tooth should be extracted no matter the age of the patient. If the tooth is severely impacted in an older pet, the client should be given the option of extraction vs. monitoring.

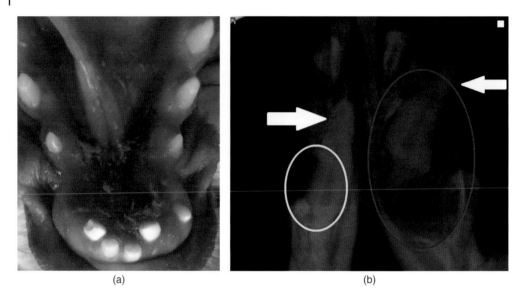

(a)   (b)

Figure 2.10 Dentigerous cyst developing on an impacted mandibular canine. (a) Intraoral dental picture of a 2-year-old dog who is "missing" the lower canines. (b) The intraoral dental radiograph of the area reveals that both canines are impacted (white arrows) and that there is a large cyst forming on the left side (red circle) and a smaller one on the right (yellow circle). All imaged teeth are malformed with short roots.

2.3.2 Sequelae

The biggest concern with unerupted or impacted teeth is the development of dentigerous cysts [21, 32] (Figure 2.10). These cysts arise from the enamel forming organ (ameloblasts) of the unerupted/impacted tooth [30]. The most common teeth to be involved with these cysts are the mandibular canine and first premolar teeth [29]. In one study, the incidence of cystic formation from impacted teeth in dogs was reported to be 29% [25]. Brachycephalic breeds are overrepresented [29].

As the cyst expands, bone is lost due to the pressure exerted by the cyst. These cysts can rapidly become quite large, resulting in an area of significantly weakened bone [12] (Figure 2.11). If this is allowed to occur, a large surgery will be required to excise the cyst. In addition, these cysts can

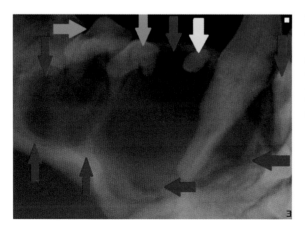

Figure 2.11 Intraoral dental radiograph of a canine patient with an impacted right mandibular first premolar (405) (yellow arrow). It has created a large dentigerous cyst (red arrows). Finally, note that the second and third premolars are being shifted distally by the pressure from the cyst (green arrows).

Figure 2.12 Intraoral dental radiograph of a canine patient with an impacted left mandibular first premolar (305) (blue arrow). It has created a large dentigerous cyst (white arrows). Finally, the pressure from the cyst has created a weakened mandible which was fractured with minimal force (red arrows). This is called a "pathologic fracture." Referral to a veterinary dentist is strongly recommended.

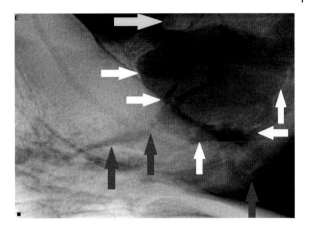

eventually result in a pathologic fracture [24, 33] (Figure 2.12). Dentigerous cysts also may become infected, thus resulting in significant discomfort for the patient [34]. Finally, these cysts are known to undergo malignant transformation [30, 35–37].

Extraction of impacted/embedded teeth requires an "open" approach, and usually bone removal to expose the tooth for extraction. If cystic formation has occurred, en bloc removal can be considered. However, most veterinary dentists will choose to extract the impacted teeth as well as any other teeth significantly affected by the cyst, followed by meticulous curettage of the lining ± bone augmentation [30, 38, 39].

If the canine teeth are impacted, the surgery will be quite challenging. This is because the apex of the tooth which is normally at the level of the mesial root of the second premolar is even further distal, often to the level of the fourth premolar (Figure 2.13). An open extraction with significant bone removal is required, and the first and second premolars often must be sacrificed to remove the impacted tooth.

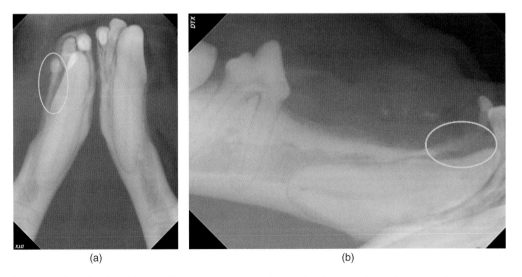

(a)   (b)

Figure 2.13 V/D (a) and lateral (b) intraoral dental radiographs of a dog with an impacted right mandibular canine (404). In addition, there is a dentigerous cyst forming around the crown (yellow circles). The apex of the root is almost back to the level of the fourth premolar, which will greatly complicate extraction. Referral to a veterinary dentist is strongly recommended.

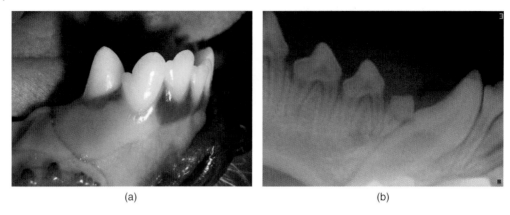

(a)   (b)

Figure 2.14 Intraoral picture (a) and dental radiograph (b) of a 16-month-old dog with an infra-erupted right mandibular canine (404). Note that the first premolar (405) is impacted, which is a common situation.

2.3.3 Infra-erupted Teeth

Infra-erupted teeth are most common in brachycephalic breeds, and small dogs are overrepresented. However, this condition can be seen in any dog. The most common teeth to be affected are the mandibular canines and first premolars, and it is occasionally seen in the mandibular first molar.

The infra-eruption results in the cervical part of the crown residing in the gingival/periodontal tissues (Figure 2.14). Since the gingiva cannot attach to the enamel, a pseudopocket is created. Pseudopockets are a convenient location for food entrapment, plaque and calculus accumulation,

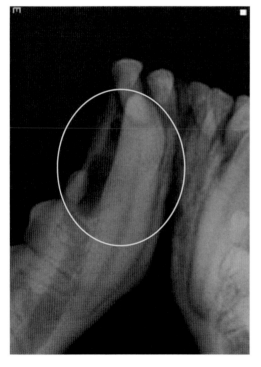

Figure 2.15 Intraoral dental radiograph of an infra-erupted right mandibular canine (404). There is a dentigerous cyst forming around the crown of the tooth (yellow circle).

and early development of periodontal disease [1, 4, 21, 40]. While rare, cystic formation may also occur (Figure 2.15).

2.3.4 Therapy

The main aim of therapy is to minimize or completely eliminate the pseudopocketing [2, 41]. If the degree of impaction is mild, a minor gingivectomy and homecare is usually sufficient [42]. If the level of impaction is such that a simple gingivectomy combined with the level of homecare provided cannot maintain the periodontal health, an apical repositioning flap is the treatment of choice [43] (Figure 2.16). This procedure lowers the gingiva to the cemento-enamel junction (CEJ) creating a normal gingival attachment and thus facilitates maintenance of periodontal health.

In severe cases, the best option is extraction, however this can be exceedingly challenging when the mandibular canines are involved. This is due to the fact that the root of the infra-erupted

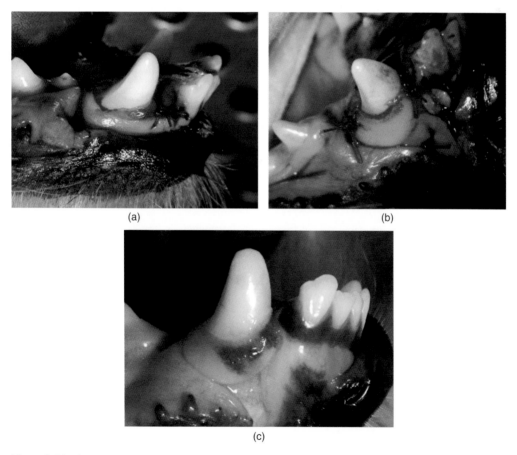

(a)　　　　(b)

(c)

Figure 2.16 A reverse bevel incision was performed, and then buccal and lingual full thickness mucogingival flaps were created with vertical releasing incisions. The ipsilateral third incisor and impacted first premolar were then extracted. The mesial incision was sutured to line up the level of the flap (a). Following correct alignment, the distal incision was sutured and finally a periosteal tacking suture placed to maintain the position of the flap. (b) Six-month recheck reveals that the flap is in proper position at the CEG and the tooth is periodontally healthy (c). Apical repositioning flap for the infra-erupted canine in Figure 2.15. For further information on this technique see the chapter Periodontal Flap Surgery in the text Veterinary Periodontology [43].

tooth is even deeper in the mandible than a normal canine (see Figure 2.13). While reported, extrusion therapy is a challenging technique requiring numerous anesthesia and is generally not recommended [31].

References

1 Wetering, A.V. (2011). Dental and oral cavity. In: *Small Animal Pediatrics* (eds. M.E. Peterson and M.A. Kutzler), 340–348. St. Louis, MO: Elsevier.

2 Startup, S. (2013). Rotated, crowded, and Supernummery teeth. In: *Veterinary Orthodontics* (ed. B.A. Niemiec), 66–72. Tustin: Practical Veterinary Publishing.

3 Hennet, P.R. and Harvey, C.E. (1992). Craniofacial development and growth in the dog. *J. Vet. Dent.* 9 (2): 11–18.

4 Hale, F.A. (2005). Juvenile veterinary dentistry. *Vet. Clin. Small Anim.* 35: 789–817.

5 Niemiec, B.A. (2013). Pathogenesis and Etiology of periodontal disease. In: *Veterinary Periodontology* (ed. B.A. Niemiec), 18–34. Ames: Wiley Blackwell.

6 Alsulaiman, A.A., Kaye, E., Jones, J. et al. (2018). Incisor malalignment and the risk of periodontal disease progression. *Am. J. Orthod. Dentofac. Orthop.* 153 (4): 512–522.

7 Debowes, L.J. (2010). Problems with the gingiva. In: *Small Animal Dental, Oral and Maxillofacial Disease, a Color Handbook* (ed. B.A. Niemiec), 159–181. London: Manson.

8 Buckley, L.A. (1972). The relationship between malocclusion and periodontal disease. *J. Periodontol.* 43 (7): 415–417.

9 Tondelli, P.M. (2019). Orthodontic treatment as an adjunct to periodontal therapy. *Dental Press J. Orthod.* 24 (4): 80–82.

10 Mitchell, P.Q. (2002). Orthodontics. In: *Small Animal Dentistry the Practical Veterinarian Series* (ed. S.P. Messonnier), 207–211. Woburn, MA: Butterworth-Heinemann.

11 Surgeon, T.W. (2005). Fundamentals of small animal orthodontics. *Vet. Clin. Small Anim.* 35: 869–889.

12 Niemiec, B.A. (2010). Pathology in the pediatric patient. In: *Small Animal Dental Oral and Maxillofacial Disease* (ed. B.A. Niemiec), 89–126. London UK: Manson.

13 Gawron, K., Łazarz-Bartyzel, K., Potempa, J., and Chomyszyn-Gajewska, M. (2016). Gingival fibromatosis: clinical, molecular and therapeutic issues. *Orphanet. J. Rare Dis.* 11: 9.

14 Blanton, P.L., Hurt, W.C., and Largent, M.D. (1977). Oral factitious injuries. *J. Periodontol.* 48 (1): 33–37.

15 Bernhardt, O., Krey, K.F., Daboul, A. et al. (2019). New insights in the link between malocclusion and periodontal disease. *J. Clin. Periodontol.* 46 (2): 144–159.

16 Startup, S. Rotated, crowded, and Supernummery teeth. In: *Veterinary Orthodontics* (ed. B.A. Niemiec). Tustin: Practical Veterinary Publishing.

17 Neville, B.W., Damm, D.D., Allen, C.M., and Bouquot, J.E. (2002). *Oral & Maxillofacial Pathology*, 2e. Philadelphia: WB Saunders.

18 Shipp, A.D. and Fahrenkrug, P. (1992). *Practitioner's Guide to Veterinary Dentistry*. Beverly Hills: Dr. Shipps Laboratories.

19 Harvey, C.E. and Emily, P.P. (1993). Function, formation, and anatomy of oral structures in carnivores. In: *Small Animal Dentistry*, 1–18. St Louis: Mosby.

20 Wiggs, R.B. and Lobprise, H.B. (1997). *Veterinary Dentistry, Principles and Practice*. Philadelphia: Lippincott-Raven.

21 Niemiec, B.A. (2010). *Pathology in the Pediatric Patient* (ed. B.A. Niemiec), 89–126. London: Manson.

22 Rossman, L.E., DADA, G., and Harvey, C.E. (1985). Disorders of teeth. In: *Veterinary Dentistry* (ed. C.E. Harvey), 79. Philadelphia: WB Saunders.

23 Lemmons, M. and Bebe, D. (2019). Oral anatomy and physiology. In: *Wiggs' Veterinary Dentistry Principals and Practice*, 2e (eds. H.B. Lobprise and J.R. Dodd), 1–24. Hoboken: Wiley Blackwell.

24 Niemiec, B.A. (2011). The importance of dental radiology. *Eur. J. Comp. Anim. Pract.* 20 (3): 219–229.

25 Babbitt, S.G., Krakowski Volker, M., and Luskin, I.R. (2016). Incidence of radiographic cystic lesions associated with unerupted teeth in dogs. *J. Vet. Dent.* 33 (4): 226–233.

26 Moore, J.I. and Niemiec, B.A. (2014). Evaluation of extraction sites for evidence of retained tooth roots and periapical pathology. *J. Am. Anim. Hosp. Assoc.* 50 (2): 77–82.

27 Shope, B.H., Mitchell, P.Q., and Carle, D. (2019). Developmental pathology and Pedodontology. In: *Wiggs' Veterinary Dentistry Principals and Practice*, 2e (eds. H.B. Lobprise and J.R. Dodd), 63–79. Hoboken: Wiley-Blackwell.

28 Carle, D. and Shope, B. (2014). Soft tissue tooth impaction in a dog. *J. Vet. Dent.* 31 (2): 96–105.

29 Verstraete, F.J., Zin, B.P., Kass, P.H. et al. (2011). Clinical signs and histologic findings in dogs with odontogenic cysts: 41 cases (1995–2010). *J. Am. Vet. Med. Assoc.* 239 (11): 1470–1476.

30 Bellows, J. (2004). Oral surgical equipment, materials, and techniques. In: *Small Animal Dental Equipment, Materials, and Techniques, a Primer*, 297–361. Blackwell.

31 Surgeon, T.W. (2000). Surgical exposure and orthodontic extrusion of an impacted canine tooth in a cat: a case report. *J. Vet. Dent.* 17 (2): 81–85.

32 Ayako, O. (2003). Dentigerous cysts in brachycephalic breed dogs and diagnostic findings and treatment with bone augmentation. *WSAVA 2003 Congress Proceedings*, Bangkok Thailand, (24–27 October 2003). pp. 121–122.

33 Niemiec, B.A. The importance of and indications for dental radiology. In: *Practical Veterinary Dental Radiology* (eds. B.A. Niemiec, J. Gawor and V. Jekel), 5–30. CRC Press.

34 Fulton, A. and Fiani, N. (2011). Diagnostic imaging in veterinary dental practice. Dentigerous cyst with secondary infection. *J. Am. Vet. Med. Assoc.* 238 (4): 435–437.

35 Neville, B.W., Damm, D.D., Allen, C.M., and Bouquot, J.E. (2002). *Oral and Maxillofacial Pathology*, 2e, 609. Philadelphia, PA: Saunders.

36 Araújo, J.P., Kowalski, L.P., Rodrigues, M.L. et al. (2014). Malignant transformation of an odontogenic cyst in a period of 10 years. *Case Rep. Dent.*: 762969.

37 Grisar, K., Schol, M., Hauben, E. et al. (2016). Primary intraosseous squamous cell carcinoma of the mandible arising from an infected odontogenic cyst: a case report and review of the literature. *Oncol. Lett.* 12 (6): 5327–5331.

38 Niemiec, B.A. (2010, 2010). Pathology in the pediatric patient. In: *Small Animal Dental, Oral and Maxillofacial Disease* (ed. B.A. Niemiec), 89–126. London: Manson.

39 Kuyama, K., Hayashi, K., Fufita, S.F. et al. (2009). Immunohistochemical analysis of a dentigerous cyst in a dog. *J. Vet. Dent.* 26 (2): 106–109.

40 DeBowes, L. (2008). Problems with the gingiva. In: *A Colour Handbook of Small Animal Oral and Maxillofacial Diseases* (ed. B.A. Niemiec), 166–194. London UK: Manson Publishing.

41 Niemiec, B.A. (2013). Gingival surgery. In: *Veterinary Periodontology* (ed. B.A. Niemiec), 193–206. Ames: Wiley Blackwell.

42 Wiggs, R.B. and Lobprise, H.B. (1997). Periodontology. In: *Veterinary Dentistry, Principles and Practice*, 186–231. Philadelphia: Lippincott-Raven.

43 Niemiec, B.A. (248, 2013). Periodontal flap surgery. In: *Veterinary Periodontology* (ed. B.A. Niemiec), 206. Ames: Wiley Blackwell.

3

The Welfare Concerns of Heritable Dental Diseases

Kymberley C. McLeod

Conundrum Consulting, Toronto, Ontario, Canada

3.1 Introduction

When considering the unique aspects of health-related welfare of small breed dogs, dental disease prevention and treatment is key to ensuring wellness. When left untreated, dogs with poor dental health may be forced to bear with significant infection, pain, emotional and/or physical distress, and even an inability to express natural behaviors [1–4]. Due to their severity, frequency, and chronicity, Summers et al. [5] determined that dental disorders create the most significant impact on overall health-related welfare, compared with other common disorders including arthritis and inflammatory skin disease. Incorporating the animal welfare impacts of dental disease in small breed patients when speaking with owners may be a challenge to some veterinarians, however advocating for the welfare of our patients must remain a core focus of veterinary medicine [6].

Due to the lack of clear visible signs, dental disease often goes unnoticed and thus unprioritized by clients. Further, understanding of the impact that dental disease can have on quality and potentially quantity of life is lacking with most pet owners (and veterinarians). Chronic disease often exists unnoticed by owners, leading to the animal suffering from the effects of their dental disease in virtual silence. Because of the acute and chronic effects on patient welfare, dental disease is an unacceptable condition for any veterinarian to leave purposefully unaddressed.

Using the central tenets of the Five Animal Welfare Needs [7] (which have evolved out of the Five Freedoms [8] to assess patient welfare), the challenges of dental conditions may be more easily evaluated and can be discussed with clients in language they can understand and embrace. Only when an owner understands, accepts, and then incorporates the necessary changes do our patients truly benefit from our wisdom.

3.2 What Is Animal Welfare?

Animal welfare has many definitions, but at its most basic level, animal welfare encompasses the physical, psychological, social, and environmental wellbeing of animals [9]. While there are parts of the world where animal welfare refers mainly to the assessment of animal cruelty or neglect, that is not the definition being utilized for this book. An animal's welfare, or its physical and emotional

Breed Predispositions to Dental and Oral Disease in Dogs, First Edition. Edited by Brook A. Niemiec.
© 2021 John Wiley & Sons, Inc. Published 2021 by John Wiley & Sons, Inc.

wellbeing, may be used somewhat interchangeably. There is increasing concern with the treatment of animals within societies around the world. Thus, allowing animals to live a life in which positive welfare is prioritized has become a mainstream topic of conversation [10]. However, deciding on what optimal welfare is or should be can be quite complex.

At the root of an animal welfare assessment lies the desire to evaluate how well an animal can cope with its environment and the challenges it faces in its daily life. Historically, there have been three main areas of focus when animal welfare issues are discussed or evaluated: health, resource/environmental, and cognitive/emotional needs [9]. While much welfare research examines only one or possibly two of these areas, ultimately the science of animal welfare encompasses all these needs.

Many people think animal welfare and the ethics of animal use are synonymous. However, animal ethics focuses on what we, as humans, think about the animal's situation based on our own morals/viewpoint, which vary widely by cultural and geographical norms [9]. An example of animal ethics might be whether an owner should be required to euthanize an animal with severe painful dental disease if they refuse to treat it. Animal welfare, in comparison, chooses to focus on the subjective needs and experience of the animal itself, i.e. what impacts on that patient's daily quality of life is the severe periodontal disease having, and what can be done to alleviate them. Dental disease poses a variety of welfare concerns due to its commonality, the wide variety of local and systemic deleterious effects, and its chronicity [11].

3.2.1 Animal Welfare Needs Assessment (AWNA)

Patient welfare exists on a spectrum. When evaluating disease, the spectrum travels from non-existent (patient has no evidence of disease) to severe (the patient is moribund). Similarly, welfare states exist from optimal (the patient's body and mental state are ideal, with all natural behaviors being possible) to minimal (all welfare needs are compromised) [12]. While a wide variety of welfare assessment methods have been developed, their use and applicability for companion animal veterinarians is somewhat challenging. However, veterinarians are excellent at assimilating information from a variety of observable sources to create a holistic conclusion on the health of a patient.

3.2.2 Introduction to the Five Freedoms/Welfare Needs

The Five Freedoms are the original basis of animal welfare assessments and considerations. They are an option to guide practicing veterinarians in conversations regarding Animal Welfare Needs Assessments (AWNAs) for un- or undertreated dental disease. Adopted and endorsed by organizations such as the World Organization for Animal Health, the Royal Society for Prevention of Cruelty to Animals (RSPCA), and the American Society for Prevention of Cruelty to Animals (ASPCA), these freedoms were first formally published by the UK Farm Animal Welfare Council [8]. They represent an ideal situation that should be strived for with each animal under care. They currently encompass: [13]

- Freedom from hunger, thirst, and malnutrition
- Freedom from pain and injury
- Freedom from infection and disease
- Freedom from fear and distress
- Freedom to express natural behaviors

While this was a wonderful start, over time the argument has been made that the idea of "freedom" from these situations, while perhaps ideal, is somewhat evolutionarily and physiologically illogical. All sentient beings experience some stress in daily life, and stressors are, in many ways, required for survival. For example, without ever experiencing the sensation of thirst, an animal wouldn't drink. Additionally, the Five Freedoms focus on the types of problems that at the time of their creation were the focus of animal welfare. While their practicality was immediately obvious for farm and research animals, both practitioners and welfare advocates found them difficult to apply to the wider range of jobs/purposes that dogs have. As such, a more meaningful and applicable approach to verbalizing these "Freedoms" was developed in 2006, and rewritten as the Five Animal Welfare Needs [14].

The Five Animal Welfare Needs are a more practitioner-friendly way of promoting and thinking about the many facets of animal's requirements in a companion animal setting. They encompass:

- The need for a suitable environment
- The need for a suitable diet
- The need to be able to exhibit normal behavior patterns
- The need to be housed with, or apart from, other animals
- The need to be protected from pain, suffering, injury, and disease

This useful framework for AWNAs acknowledges the strengths of what the Five Freedoms had achieved. However, in order to encourage conversation around the importance of understanding, identifying, and minimizing negative welfare states, the Five Animal Welfare Needs are worded in a more proactive way. By ensuring our clients understand what it means to provide a healthy environment, appropriate behavioral expression opportunities, optimal nutrition, excellent health, and positive mental experiences, we can positively guide the way our clients care for their animals, and potentially choose breeding stock free from heritable dental conditions.

Evaluation and discussion of a small or toy breed dog's current, and potentially predictable future welfare needs should be part of every veterinary exam. Appropriate client communication and information gathering, clinical assessment, and behavioral observations, along with the physical exam findings all help to identify potential welfare shortcomings [15]. Maintaining and improving the welfare of our small and "at risk" patients also requires regular factual recording of AWNAs within the patient file, including both the pet's physical and emotional welfare. The Five Welfare Needs basis for AWNA allows a practitioner to approach and evaluate physical and psychological wellbeing in a practical and approachable manner and is already regularly being utilized in the UK [14].

3.2.3 Dental Diseases Compromise Patient Welfare

In the past, it was a generally held belief that dogs didn't need dental care, and that bad breath and even tooth loss was a minor issue with little consequence to health. However, recent studies have shown that due to their severity, frequency, and chronicity in dogs, dental disorders have the most significant impact on overall health-related welfare [11]. Diseases of the oral cavity and teeth are some of the most common medical conditions in small and toy breed dogs [16–22]. A significant number of veterinary patients are dealing with pain, infection, or both on a daily basis.

3.2.4 Periodontal Disease in Small Breed Dogs

Small breed dogs (under 10 kg), Greyhounds, and Cavalier King Charles Spaniels, experience a far greater prevalence and severity of periodontal disease compared to their larger equivalents

[16–20, 23] (see Chapter 1). Tooth crowding, increased retention of deciduous teeth due to improper eruption path of the permanent teeth, and resultant redundant dentition and mal-occlusions are the result of genetic selection for smaller dogs and/or abnormal head shape [24]. The abnormal gingival attachment that results, along with increased food entrapment which encourages periodontal bacteria to flourish, hastens the development of periodontal disease [25–27]. Unlike larger breeds, small breed dogs are significantly more likely to develop periodontal disease, including 30% of dogs under 10 lb showing bone loss by the age of 12 months [28]. When veterinarians treat all dogs like the most robust large breed example, diagnosis and therapy of periodontal issues is significantly delayed. This leads to breeds which are predisposed to periodontal issues at younger ages experiencing more advanced disease without therapy for longer stretches. Allowing the pain and infection of advanced periodontal disease to go untreated due to ignorance is a significant welfare concern. All predisposed breeds should have regular therapy beginning early in life, to ensure health and welfare are maximized.

3.3 Sequelae to Periodontal Disease

Small breed dogs are also much more likely to develop severe local sequelae to their periodontal disease when compared to medium and large breed dogs. All small breed dogs are prone to oronasal fistulas, experiencing them at far higher rates [29–31]. Dolichocephalic breeds, such as Dachshunds, struggle with oronasal fistulas most frequently, and may experience pain and nasal discharge due to chronic sinusitis for extended periods because of misdiagnosis. Many animals with oronasal fistulas have relatively clean crowns and minimal gingivitis, therefore a thorough probing of the maxillary teeth should be performed regularly on all predisposed breeds from an early age [32]. Additionally, animals showing suspicious nasal symptoms should also receive an anesthetized dental exam before more advanced imaging is done, to expedite diagnosis of the oronasal fistula (see Chapter 1).

As breeders selected for smaller frame sizes, the skeletal system shrunk more rapidly than the dental elements, resulting in dogs with proportionally large teeth in relatively delicate jaws [33, 34]. Many breeds under 10 kg exhibit extraordinarily thin mandibles compared to the size of the cheek teeth. Normal dogs from many of these small breeds may only have millimeters of bone surrounding their mandibular canines, premolars, and molars. Sadly, these breeds are also more prone to the apical infection and bone lysis of progressive periodontal disease. This combination can be disastrous, resulting in further loss of mandibular integrity and eventually, pathologic fracture. The smaller the breed, the more likely the pathologic fracture. Pathological fractures can occur organically, from play or fighting with other dogs, or with application of force while cleaning or extracting teeth. When performing a professional dental cleaning on a small breed dog, dental radiology is essential to assess the health of the mandible and plan appropriate treatment. If a practitioner is unable to x-ray the mouth, or upon radiographic examination feels a pathologic fracture may occur during therapy, referral must be offered to the owner [35]. If the owner decides to move forward with therapy, informed consent includes discussion of the risks of fracture and its appropriate treatment, along with the benefits to the animal of therapy. Ethically, we must be self-aware and report to the owners our level of competency under these circumstances, as well as our access to all necessary equipment (see Chapter 11).

3.4   Gingival Hyperplasia

Genetically induced gingival hyperplasia is mainly seen in Boxers, but also Dobermans and St. Bernards have been noted to be affected [36, 37]. While its etiology is unknown, this increase in gingival tissue leads to excessive pocketing and an increased rate of periodontal colonization [24, 37–39]. Like other situations where periodontal disease occurs, the pain and physiological drain from infection due to this condition must not be minimized or overlooked (see Chapter 7).

3.5   Associations with Pain and Suffering

When assessing patients with dental disease using the FAWN system, the majority of focus is placed on the need to be protected from pain, suffering, injury, and disease, as well as the need to be able to exhibit normal behavior patterns.

The International Association for the Study of Pain (ISAP) defines pain as "an unpleasant sensory and emotional experience associated with actual or potential tissue damage or described in terms of such damage" [40]. The human literature describes dental pain as extreme due to amount of innervation within the tooth and jaw [41, 42]. Decreased productivity, sleep disturbance, and notable social and psychological impacts can all be seen when humans experience chronic dental pain or infection [43–45]. However, pain is an experience unique to the individual, and predictable behaviors associated with pain are very species-specific [46–49]. This is in large part due to the variation in number, distribution, and morphology of opioid receptors [50].

There are few behaviors in dogs one can reliably link to oral pain reported in the literature. This is likely the reason that many within the veterinary profession don't feel dental disease is or could be painful. It is important to note that despite the apparent lack of behavioral indicators, an animal's experience of dental pain and infection is likely to be equally present [46, 51], given that oral innervation and pain thresholds of people and dogs are quite similar [52, 53].

To illustrate this more definitively, non-human mammals have been found to be excellent models for dental pain in the human world [46, 54, 55]. Prolifically utilized in nociception and pain relief pharmaceutical research, small rodents are an excellent model for pulpitis, which causes extreme pain responses in humans. Repeatable and measurable behavioral changes from pulpal pain in rodents include increased time to complete meals, shaking, weight loss and/or decreased growth rates, open-mouthed yawns, freezing, and overall decreased activity [46, 49]. Dogs and cats have also been utilized to show behavioral changes with pulpal and non-pulpal pain [54, 55]. It is interesting to note that despite the common belief amongst veterinary professionals and owners alike that dental pain will lead to a dramatic decrease or total cessation of appetite, this has rarely been noted in the published research [56].

While we cannot always prove an animal is in pain, the veterinary profession must seek to relieve pain we *suspect* in our patients under all circumstances [57, 58]. Owner understanding of the changes that generalized chronic pain may cause in their companion animals is mixed, and varies greatly in its predictive ability for recognition [59–61].

Effective therapy is justified and should be started immediately to alleviate suspected oral pain upon diagnosis of oral disease [57]. Pain cannot be proven to be present or absent based on oral examination, radiographs, or CT. While temporary measures may be possible with observable improvements with the use of pharmaceuticals [62, 63], the only way to remove pain definitively is to address the issue with appropriate and complete dental therapy, which almost always requires general anesthesia.

3.6 Physiological Signs of Stress

Within an AWNA, a stressor is defined as any event that alters homeostatic equilibrium and therefore necessitates adaptation to reestablish natural homeostasis. The physiological disturbances caused by stressors create a state of physiological stress, which may lead to suffering and/or mental distress [64]. Endodontic and periodontal disease caused by infectious etiologies also incur a significant bacterial disease burden on the body [65–68].

Potentially deleterious consequences come from the unrelenting pain and infection as the body's natural stress responses are activated [69]. Acute stressors stimulate the sympathetic nervous system to immediately release adrenaline and noradrenaline, leading to behavioral and physical responses. Over time, the longer acting hypothalamic-pituitary-adrenal (HPA) axis may become stimulated, causing a more chronic cortisol release within the system.

Physical stimulation of a complicated fracture in a conscious animal may create observable responses from this system, such as attempts to escape. Other potential responses include vocalization, increased heart rate, trembling, and release of blood glucose in preparation to fight or flee. Long-standing stimulation, such as from severe periodontal disease that results in an oronasal fistula, may lead to chronic inflammatory stimulation of the HPA axis. Chronic infectious or inflammatory stressors negatively affect multiple body systems. Immune function impacts may be first noted with the development of an acute stress leukogram, progressing to leukopenia and immunosuppressive inflammatory cytokine changes with chronicity. Chronic stress responses have also been linked to decreased ability to eliminate bacterial infection and increased susceptibility to disease in humans and mice [70–72]. Untreated dental disease can lead to chronic inflammation and infection of the oral tissues [73, 74]. Unchecked or chronic infection is ethically unacceptable to leave without recommendation of appropriate therapy [69].

3.6.1 Behavior Changes Noted with Physiological Stress and Pain

Behavioral scoring systems to evaluate pain exist for a variety of systems and species [75, 76]. It is important to note, however, that dental pain indicators are often vague and non-specific. Oral conditions generally recognized to be painful include periodontal disease, tooth and jaw fractures, tooth resorption, caries, caudal stomatitis, traumatic malocclusions, and some oral neoplasias. The absence of a notable behavioral change does not signify a lack of pain, nor does it imply any lack of severity. Dogs may simply not show the pain they are enduring chronically in an easily observable or understandable way to their owners or veterinarians [77]. Pain behaviors that have been well attributed to dental pain in dogs include drooling, repetitive licking, mutilation of the mouth, pawing, rubbing, and slightly decreased appetite [78–80].

A common argument against the supposition that dental diseases are painful and debilitating is to point out that dogs will continue to consume food in the face of severe disease. Animals require nourishment to survive, and the instinct to survive is stronger than the desire to avoid pain [81a]. Another common argument is that dogs may continue demonstrating normal oral behaviors, such as playing with toys and using their mouth to explore their environment despite experiencing dental pain. Many people continue to perform crucial and non crucial activities despite chronic pain. It is not uncommon for people to continue working or playing sports despite debilitating conditions such as arthritis or migraine headaches. Dogs with other chronically painful conditions, such as osteoarthritis, also show continuation of many normal play behaviours despite the influence of the discomfort of their condition [81b]. While not all animals show decreased play, anecdotally owners report feeling their animals are prevented from expressing these natural and essential behaviors due to chronic discomfort, which also reduces their overall welfare [80]. Additionally, clients report that they are happier to know their pets are not in pain [82a,b]. Regardless of change in behavior, the underlying pain should not be a condition which the animal is expected to endure, either by the veterinary community or by owners [69].

3.6.2 Client Educational Goals

As veterinarians, it is our responsibility to proactively diagnose, treat, and relieve pain and suffering for our animal patients. Additional education may help clients understand the decreased welfare associated with dental disease, and it may assist in increasing compliance with the recommended treatment plan. To allow untreated dental disease to cause continuous pain without therapy is a significant animal welfare issue [83].

A simple questionnaire or discussion during regular health exams regarding current oral and facial behaviors as well as any changes to oral odor, should be performed and recorded in the patient's medical record. While anecdotally it appears that most owners and many veterinarians feel oral pain will decrease appetite (and therefore in its absence lead to misreported changes), we encourage practitioners to consider a more universal view to the wide variety of changes that may be noted as sequelae to oral disease [80]. It is important that the veterinarian not ask leading or closed-ended questions, but have the owner to evaluate any changes they may have noticed regarding these issues. Equally important is to enquire about any additional positive or negative changes the owner has noted since professional dental therapy has been completed. Contacting the owner approximately two- and eight-weeks post-therapy is commonly advised, to get a full picture of the improvements noted following therapy.

3.6.3 Welfare Issues Surrounding the Veterinary Dental Visit, Handling Techniques, and Procedural Design

The welfare needs of our patients during a veterinary visit begin from the time they are being prepared to leave their home to when they return and have completed healing from their dental procedure. The importance of evaluating the welfare needs of our patients is universally important medically, even if educational and socioeconomic levels, standards of care, availability of resources, and societal demands may vary around the world [83]. Additionally, negative experiences during veterinary hospital visits can quickly disrupt the tenuous human: animal bond and also decrease a client's bond with and trust in the veterinary hospital team [84–86].

As sentient beings, our companion animals have the ability to experience not just pain and distress, but both positive (pleasure, comfort, stimulatory) and negative (fear, anxiety) emotions [87]. At all times when working with our veterinary patients, the aim should be to prevent fear, anxiety, and stress (FAS), and a patients' level of FAS should be assessed and considered at each step of the dental patient experience [88–91]. Multimodal approaches can help offset the variation in individual response to each method of stress reduction, and should be employed wherever possible [92, 93].

Fear, anxiety and/or pain leads to stimulation of the SNS and the HPA axis [94]. Adverse experiences may stimulate the fight-flight-freeze reaction, and possibly create aggressive behavior while being handled as well as during subsequent visits. Chronic stimulation can decrease immune function, extend healing times, or even cause breakdown of surgical closure [64]. Stress experienced by the patient during veterinary care may also contribute to higher doses of anesthesia and analgesia

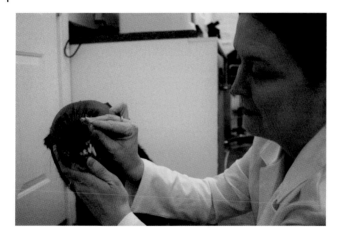

Figure 3.1 Appropriate low stress oral exam on a canine patient. In general, exam gloves should be worn, but in some cases, they can be very disturbing to the patient. Approach the patient slowly but confidently. Do not force the exam on an unwilling patient. Consider blocking visual stimulus with an opaque eye covering to reduce patient reactivity.

being required to maintain an adequate anesthetic plane, with potentially increased adverse anesthetic outcomes [95, 96]. Stressors sensitize the central nervous system and increase reactivity due to repeated stimulation of C-fiber nociceptors, leading to central spinal neuron sensitization. The increase in intensity of perceived pain, and resultant physiological and physical responses from the animal are known as "wind-up pain" [97]. Also associated with "wind-up pain" is an increased difficulty to manage pain post-surgically [98].

Travel to and from the veterinary hospital is the first area that may increase FAS [99]. Educating clients on techniques to reduce physiological stress during transport so that our patients arrive at the hospital at the lowest stimulation level possible is the first step [100, 101]. Early and frequent socialization of small breed dogs to travel, utilizing a clean carrier that is the appropriate size for a small dog, pheromone diffusers or sprays [102], and pharmacological options to address stress and anxiety can all assist in reducing the negative effects of travel [103].

All dental assessment and therapy must be provided by properly trained veterinary professionals. Gentle, respectful handling improves the patient's experience and memory of the event, but has also been shown to improve post-operative healing and decrease anesthetic need [92, 104, 105]. During initial oral examination, handling techniques to allow for less stress of the patient should be utilized [92] (Figure 3.1). The use of anxiolytics therapeutically for reduction of anxiety or stress is highly encouraged where appropriate [106]. Prevention of pain and stress at the time of initial exam may prevent creation of negative behavioral outcomes at future visits that make oral examination more difficult [107]. Education on, and commitment to reducing stress involved with handling for oral exams and procedures related to dental therapy is essential when addressing dental disease in our patients. If reasonable, gentle handling techniques are unsuccessful to allow for examination, suitable sedation or antianxiety medications must be considered [106] (Figure 3.2). Punishment, rough, and/or dominant handling techniques have no place in the veterinary hospital and must be eradicated [92, 108, 109].

Once the veterinary healthcare professional has conducted an appropriate and thorough oral exam, any pathology noted must be communicated to the client, and an appropriate treatment plan recommended to resolve the issues noted. Lack of intervention in the face of dental disease contributes to continued negative welfare implications for our patients, and thus, a decreased level of wellbeing. When appropriate therapy is available, it must be recommended and advocated for.

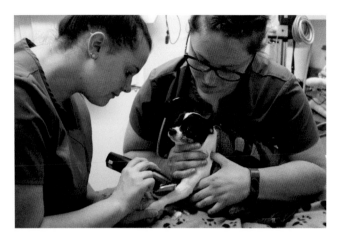

Figure 3.2   Gentle handling should be used at all times. If a small breed struggles, it can cause injury and make future visits more challenging. In addition, it can affect oxygenation (especially in brachycephalic breeds). Appropriate sedation should always be provided.

Without excellent communication and advocacy, clients may not understand the urgency or importance of addressing the dental issue.

Reduction of the amount of stress a patient experiences during a dental procedure starts with conscientious hospital design. Waiting room design [105, 110, 111], and thoughtful patient placement while inside the hospital awaiting surgery or recovering, can reduce the amount of stress a small dog experiences while in the hospital for a dental procedure [91, 112, 113]. Anxious patients may benefit from being isolated in areas that reduce the amount of auditory and visual stimulus, and the utilization of white noise or species specific music in the hospital [114] have been shown to offset stress in some patients, while other dogs may prefer to wait with their owner outside the clinic before a procedure. Use of species appropriate pheromones upon admission (on towels placed over carriers, on treated bandanas, and as diffusers in kennel areas), and administering anxiety relieving pre-medications as soon as possible may also help [115] (Figure 3.3a).

Pre-anesthetic fasting recommendations have changed greatly in the last decade. Recent studies have shown that consumption of small amounts of easily digested liquid-based nutrition does not worsen regurgitation or anesthetic risk, and may even reduce it [116–118]. Utilization of carefully

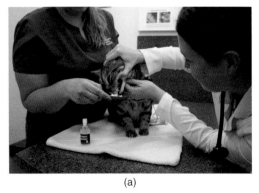

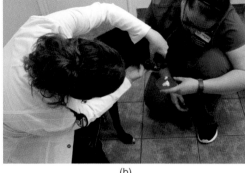

(a)   (b)

Figure 3.3   Using pheromones (a) and soft treats for distraction (a & b) can greatly ease the oral exam and procedure. These should be utilized in addition to other pharmacologic options to facilitate the experience.

selected "treats," such as frozen chicken broth cubes or a small amount of soft pate or canned food a patient can lick, can distract patients from unpleasant sensations like IV catheter placement, and encourage good behavior (Figure 3.3b). Smearing a highly desired substance within a small space (disposable cup, washable dog toy with an empty center, etc.) can extend the amount of time an animal is distracted by the food reward.

Finally, anticipating where pain may occur during each step of a professional cleaning, and reducing conscious perception of this pain will reduce "windup pain" and its deleterious effects. The use of topical anesthetic applied to IV sites prior to insertion has been very promising, and dental blocks for all extraction and surgical sites must be utilized. Gentle, efficient, and thoughtful tissue handling (minimally invasive surgery) is recommended to prevent excessive pain and swelling post-procedure [119–122]. Mouth gag use is associated with negative outcomes including blindness, and avoidance of their use is highly recommended, especially in cats [123, 124].

Local and regional anesthetic blocks and adequate pre- and post-operative pain management, are not optional. Dental surgical procedures cause predictable pain and inflammation and must be addressed to prevent excessive suffering after anesthetic recovery [81a]. Animals experiencing acute and unaddressed pain post-procedure have extended healing times and higher physiological stress levels than those whose pain is adequately addressed [81a]. Post-operative pain assessment using behavior or grimace models should be done multiple times in the period following a professional dental cleaning, and again before discharge from the hospital, with additional pain medication to be used at home until it can be reasonably anticipated it is no longer needed.

3.7 Welfare Implications of Anesthesia Free Dentistry (AFD)

Dental procedures or cleanings performed without anesthesia, commonly known as anesthesia-free dentistry (AFD) or non-anesthetic dentistry (NAD), holds no medical benefit to the animal [83]. Predictable and preventable pain, anxiety and stress must be addressed during veterinary care for both moral and ethical reasons. There are multiple aspects of a complete professional dental cleaning and oral assessment that, if done without adequate pain and anxiety relief, would create significant negative animal welfare outcomes, and concern for overall patient wellbeing.

Determining the health of gingival and subgingival tissue requires thorough periodontal probing [125–128]. It is exceedingly challenging to perform accurate probing of all surfaces of the tooth, especially the lingual/palatal surfaces and the caudal teeth, on an awake animal. Head movement and tongue interference in a conscious patient, decreased lighting, and difficulty visualizing the probe markings all contribute as reasons a conscious exam is likely to be inaccurate. While this may be a procedure that creates minimal pain in healthy individuals, probing diseased tissues such as resorptive lesions elicits a significant and predictable pain response. Determining which animals will experience pain or be stressed by the restraint required to do an awake periodontal probing is rarely accurate, and as such, a practitioner has little ability to ensure the process will not be deleterious to patient welfare [125].

Dental cleaning in the awake patient does not allow for radiological examination of the subgingival anatomy. Without effective radiographic evaluation of the dentition, significant pathology may be missed up to 40% of the time, and thus therapeutic treatment will not be delivered to the patient [129–132].

The positioning required to accurately assess all areas of the mouth and perform a thorough scaling and polishing of the teeth demands extended time in potentially stressful and compromising body positions for the patient. High velocity water sprays, and physical removal of infectious debris within the oral cavity while in these positions without protection of the airways increases potential for aspiration pneumonia [125, 133, 134]. Scaling and polishing teeth with gingival recession, resorptive lesions, or fractures may cause unnecessary pain to the conscious patient.

Scaling and polishing the visible surfaces of the teeth often leads to a cosmetically clean oral cavity with persistent infection, inflammation, and pain under the gumline [125]. Therefore, not only is the procedure potentially ineffective for removing pain and infection, it often results in a false sense of therapeutic benefit for the owner (and practitioner), which may lead to delays in appropriate care for the animal. It is ethically unacceptable to perform a mainly cosmetic procedure and leave painful and/or infectious disease [83].

The intensity of handling and restraint required for a thorough dental evaluation in a conscious patient is increased in small breed dogs, especially toy breeds under 5 kg. This adds in a layer of complexity to the situation due to their exceedingly small size. Traditionally recognized as more challenging to handle with higher levels of negative behavioral responses in the veterinary hospital, toy breed dogs may struggle and move more than their larger counterparts, and exhibit more stranger aggression [4, 135]. Lack of socialization at an early age, more frequent carrying by the owner, and different breed-based temperaments and levels of anxiety due to handling may contribute to a more difficult awake evaluation. Additionally, with their higher likelihood of periodontal disease and bone loss, jaw fracture risk becomes higher due to increased jaw fragility.

The stress and/or discomfort incurred by time consuming cosmetic procedures are both wholly avoidable by utilizing appropriate anesthesia, and indefensible from a medical and ethical standpoint. The reason for providing humane and appropriate dental care is to improve patient welfare, wellbeing, and quality of life. As such, the practice of veterinary dental procedures without appropriate anesthesia must stop. It is inadequate and provides a substandard level of care which may be misleading to the pet owner. This statement has been echoed by multiple local, national, and international veterinary medical organizations and specialty colleges of veterinary dentistry [83].

3.8 Conclusions

As advocates of humane animal husbandry and veterinary care, the veterinary profession is called to continuously improve and safeguard the welfare of our patients. We must continue to voice the need for proper dental care for our patients, advocate for optimal oral health, and educate our clients on the importance of quality dental care to the daily welfare of their pets. By utilizing the Five Animal Welfare Needs as our guide, regular dental examination and proper therapy will help to address infection, control pain, relieve suffering, allow return to regular behavior, and ultimately improve the daily welfare of our patients.

References

1 Trowbridge, H.O., Syngcuk, K., and Hideaki, S. (2002). Structure and functions of the dentin-pulp complex. In: *Pathways of the Pulp*, 8e (eds. S. Cohen and R.C. Burns), 411–456. St. Louis, MO: Mosby.

2 Niemiec, B.A. (2013). Understanding the disease process. In: *Veterinary Periodontology* (ed. B.A. Niemiec), 18–34. Ames: Wiley Blackwell.

3 Palmeira, M.I., de Oliveira, J.T., and Requicha, J.F. (2017). Dental diseases and pain in cats (*Felis catus*). *Proceedings of the 25th European Congress of Veterinary Dentistry*, Dublin (19–22 May 2016). European Veterinary Society.

4 McGreevy, P.D., Georgevsky, D., Carrasco, J. et al. (2013). Dog behavior co-varies with height, bodyweight and skull shape. *PLoS One* 8 (12): e80529. https://doi.org/10.1371/journal.pone.0080529.

5 Summers, J.F., O'Neill, D.G., Church, D. et al. (2019). Health-related welfare prioritisation of canine disorders using electronic health records in primary care practice in the UK. *BMC Vet. Res.* 15 (1): 163. https://doi.org/10.1186/s12917-019-1902-0.

6 Paul, E. and Podberscek, A. (2000). Veterinary education and students' attitudes towards animal welfare. *Vet. Rec.* 146 (10): 269–272.

7 Ryan, S., Bacon, H., Endenburg, N. et al. (2019). WSAVA animal welfare guidelines. *J. Small Anim. Pract.* 60: E1–E46. https://doi.org/10.1111/jsap.12998.

8 Brambell, R. (1965). *Report of the Technical Committee to Enquire into the Welfare of Animals Kept Under Intensive Livestock Husbandry Systems, Cmd.* (Great Britain: Parliament), 1–84. H.M. Stationery Office.

9 Palmer, C. and Sandoe, P. (2018). Animal ethics. In: *Animal Welfare*, 3e (eds. M.C. Appleby et al.), 3–15. CABI.

10 Siegford, J., Cottee, S., and Widowski, T. (2010). Opportunities for learning about animal welfare from online courses to graduate degrees. *J. Vet. Med. Educ.* 37 (1): 49–55.

11 Summers, J.F., O'Neill, D.G., Church, D. et al. (2019). Health-related welfare prioritization of canine disorders using electronic health records in primary care practice in the UK. *BMC Vet. Res.* 15 (1): 163. https://doi.org/10.1186/s12917-019-1902-0.

12 Hewson, C.J. (2003). What is animal welfare? Common definitions and their practical consequences. *Can. Vet. J.* 44: 496–499.

13 National Archives (2018). Farm animal welfare council – 5 freedoms. http://webarchive.nationalarchives.gov.uk/20121010012427/www.fawc.org.uk/freedoms.htm (accessed 18 June 2020).

14 PDSA (2018). Your pet's 5 welfare needs. www.pdsa.org.uk/taking-care-of-your-pet/looking-after-your-pet/all-pets/5-welfare-needs (accessed 18 June 2020).

15 Hewson, C.J., Wojciechowska, J.I., Patronek, G.J. et al. (2003). But is she suffering? Novel instrument to assess quality of life of pet dogs. *Anim. Welf.* 2003.

16 Hoffmann, T.H. and Gaengler, P. (1996). Clinical and pathomorphological investigation of spontaneously occurring periodontal disease in dogs. *J. Small Anim. Pract.* 37: 471–479.

17 Hamp, S.E., Hamp, M., Olsson, S.E. et al. (1997). Radiography of spontaneous periodontitis in dogs. *J. Periodontal. Res.* 32 (7): 589–597.

18 Bauer, A.E., Stella, J., Lemmons, M., and Croney, C.C. (2018). Evaluating the validity and reliability of a visual dental scale for detection of periodontal disease (PD) in non-anesthetized dogs (*Canis familiaris*). *PLoS One* 13 (9): e0203930.

19 O'Neill, D.G., Ballantyne, Z.F., Hendricks, A. et al. (2019). West Highland White Terriers under primary veterinary care in the UK in 2016: demography, mortality and disorders. *Canine Genet. Epidemiol.* 6: 7.

20 Wallis, C., Pesci, I., Colyer, A. et al. (2019). A longitudinal assessment of periodontal disease in Yorkshire terriers. *BMC Vet. Res.* 15 (1): 207.

21 Bellows, J. (2004). Equipping the dental practice. In: *Small Animal Dental Equipment, Materials, and Techniques, a Primer*, 13–55. Blackwell.

22 Niemiec, B.A. (2012). Etiology and pathogenesis of periodontal disease. In: *Veterinary Periodontology* (ed. B.A. Niemiec), 18–34. Ames: Wiley.

23 O'Neill, D.G., Rooney, N.J., Brock, C. et al. (2019). Greyhounds under general veterinary care in the UK during 2016: demography and common disorders. *Canine Genet. Epidemiol.* 6: 4.

24 Wetering, A.V. (2011). Dental and oral cavity. In: *Small Animal Pediatrics* (eds. M.E. Peterson and M.A. Kutzler), 340–348. St. Louis, MO: Elsevier.

25 Mitchell, P.Q. (2002). Orthodontics. In: *Small Animal Dentistry*, The Practical Veterinarian Series (ed. S.P. Messonnier), 207–211. Woburn, MA: Butterworth–Heinemann.

26 Surgeon, T.W. (2005). Fundamentals of small animal orthodontics. *Vet. Clin. North Am. Small Anim. Prac.* Elsevier, St Louis, MO 35: 869–889.

27 Startup, S. (2013). Rotated, crowded, and supernummery teeth. In: *Veterinary Orthodontics* (ed. B.A. Niemiec), 66–72. Tustin: Practical Veterinary Publishing.

28 Queck, K. (2018). Oral-fluid thiol-detection test identifies underlying active periodontal disease not detected by the visual awake examination. *JAAHA* 54 (3): 132–137.

29 Holmstrom, S.E., Frost, P., and Eisner, E.R. (1998). Exodontics. In: *Veterinary Dental Techniques*, 2e, 215–224. Philadelphia, PA: Saunders.

30 Niemiec, B.A. (2010). Pathologies of the oral mucosa. In: *Small Animal Dental, Oral, and Maxillofacial Disease, a Color Handbook* (ed. B.A. Niemiec), 183–198. London: Manson.

31 Niemiec, B.A. (2012). Local and regional consequences of periodontal disease. In: *Veterinary Periodontology* (ed. B.A. Niemiec), 69–80. Ames: Wiley.

32 Niemiec, B.A. (2008). Periodontal disease. *Top. Companion Anim. Med.* 23 (2): 72–80.

33 Gioso, M.A., Shofer, F., Barros, P.S., and Harvery, C.E. Mandible and mandibular first molar tooth measurements in dogs: relationship of radiographic height to body weight. *J. Vet. Dent.* 18 (2): 65–68.

34 Mulligan, T., Aller, S., and Williams, C. (1998). *Atlas of Canine and Feline Dental Radiography*, 176–183. Trenton, NJ: Veterinary Learning Systems.

35 AAHA (2013). AAHA referral and consultation guidelines. www.aaha.org/globalassets/02-guidelines/referral/aaha-referral-guidelines-2013 (accessed 18 June 2020).

36 Burstone, M.S., Bond, E., and Litt, C.R. (1952). Familial gingival hypertrophy in the dog (boxer breed). *AMA Arch. Pathol.* 54 (2): 208–212.

37 DeBowes, L. (2008). Problems with the gingiva. In: *A Colour Handbook of Small Animal Oral and Maxillofacial Diseases* (ed. B.A. Niemiec), 166–194. London: Manson Publishing.

38 Niemiec, B.A. (2010). *Pathology in the Pediatric Patient* (ed. B.A. Niemiec), 89–126. London: Manson.

39 Hale, F.A. (2005). Juvenile veterinary dentistry. *Vet. Clin. Small Anim.* Elsevier, St Louis MO 35: 789–817.

40 Merskey, H. and Bogduk, N. (1994). *Classification of Chronic Pain: Descriptions of Chronic Pain Syndromes and Definitions of Pain Terms*, 210. Seattle: International Association for the Study of Pain Press.

41 Bender, I.B. (2000). Pulpal pain diagnosis: a review. *J. Endod.* 26: 175–179.

42 Hargreaves, K.M. and Kaiser, K. (2004). New advances in the management of endodontic pain emergencies. *J. Calif. Dent. Assoc.* 32: 469–473.

43 Anil, S., Anil, L., and Deen, J. (2002). Challenges of pain assessment in domestic animals. *J. Am. Vet. Med. Assoc.* 220: 313–319. https://doi.org/10.2460/javma.2002.220.313.

44 Heaivilin, N., Gerbert, B., Page, J.E., and Gibbs, J.L. (2011). Public health surveillance of dental pain via Twitter. *J. Dent. Res.* 90 (9): 1047–1051.

45 Choi, J.W., Choi, Y., Lee, T. et al. (2019). Employment status and unmet dental care needs in South Korea: a population-based panel study. *BMJ Open* 9 (3): e022436.

46 Chidiac, J.J., Rifai, K., Hawwa, N.N. et al. (2002). Nociceptive behaviour induced by dental application of irritants to rat incisors: a new model for tooth inflammatory pain. *Eur. J. Pain* 6: 55–67.

47 Paul-Murphy, J., Ludders, J., Robertson, S. et al. (2004). The need for a cross-species approach to the study of pain in animals. *J. Am. Vet. Med. Assoc.* 224 (5): 692–697.

48 Seksel, K. (2007). How pain affects animals. Proceedings of the Australian Animal Welfare Strategy Science Summit on Pain and Pain Management. Melbourne, Australia (18 May 2007). Canberra: AAWS.

49 Chudler, E.H. and Byers, M.R. (2005). Behavioural responses following tooth injury in rats. *Arch. Oral Biol.* 50: 333–340.

50 Landau, R. (2006). One size does not fit all: genetic variability of mu-opioid receptor and post-operative morphine consumption. *Anesthesiology* 105 (2): 235–237.

51 Cohen, A.S. and Brown, D.C. (2002). Orofacial dental pain emergencies: endodontic diagnosis and management. In: *Pathways of the Pulp*, 8e (eds. A.S. Cohen and R.C. Burns), 31–76. St. Louis, MO: Mosby.

52 Bennett, G.J. and Xie, Y.K. (1988). A peripheral mononeuropathy in rat that produces disorders of pain sensation like those seen in man. *Pain* 33 (1): 87–107.

53 Rollin, B. (1989). *The Unheeded Cry: Animal Consciousness, Animal Pain, and Science*, vol. xii, 117–118. New York, NY: Oxford University Press.

54 Ahlberg, K.F. (1978). Dose-dependent inhibition of sensory nerve activity in the feline dental pulp by anti-inflammatory drugs. *Acta Physiol. Scand.* 102: 434–440.

55 Le Bars, D., Gozariu, M., and Cadden, S.W. (2001). Animal models of nociception. *Pharmacol. Rev.* 53 (4): 597–652.

56 Evangelista, M.C., Watanabe, R., Leung, V.S.Y. et al. (2019). Facial expressions of pain in cats: the development and validation of a Feline Grimace Scale. *Sci. Rep.* 9: 19128.

57 Mathews, K., Kronen, P.W., Lascelles, D. et al. (2014). Guidelines for recognition, assessment and treatment of pain. *J. Small. Anim. Pract.* 55: E10–E68.

58 Olsson, A., Wurbel, H., and Mench, J. (2018). Behaviour. In: *Animal Welfare*, 3e (eds. M.C. Appleby et al.), 3–15. CABI.

59 Yazbek, K.V. and Fantoni, D.T. (2005). Validity of a health-related quality-of-life scale for dogs with signs of pain secondary to cancer. *J. Am. Vet. Med. Assoc.* 226: 1354–1358.

60 Budke, C.M., Levine, J.M., Kerwin, S.C. et al. (2008). Evaluation of a questionnaire for obtaining owner-perceived, weighted quality-of-life assessments for dogs with spinal cord injuries. *J. Am. Vet. Med. Assoc.* 233: 925–930.

61 Wojciechowska, J.I., Hewson, C.J., Stryhn, H. et al. (2005). Evaluation of a questionnaire regarding nonphysical aspects of quality of life in sick and healthy dogs. *Am. J. Vet. Res.* 66: 1461–1467.

62 Bennett, D. and Morton, C. (2009). A study of owner observed behavioural and lifestyle changes in cats with musculoskeletal disease before and after analgesic therapy. *J. Feline Med. Surg.* 11: 997–1004.

63 Benito-de-la-Vibora, J., Gruen, M.E., Thomson, A. et al. (2012). Owner-assessed indices of quality of life in cats and the relationship to the presence of degenerative joint disease. *J. Feline Med. Surg.* 14: 863–870.

64 Moberg, G. (2000). Biological response to stress: implications for animal welfare. In: *The Biology of Animal Stress: Basic Principles and Implications for Animal Welfare* (eds. G.P. Moberg and J.A. Mench), 1–21. CABI.

65 DeBowes, L.J. (1996). The effects of dental disease on systemic disease. *Vet. Clin. North Am. Small Anim. Pract.* 28 (5): 1057–1062.

66 Scannapieco, F.A. (2004). Periodontal inflammation: from gingivitis to systemic disease? *Compend. Contin. Educ. Dent.* 25 (Suppl 1): 16–25.

67 Mealy, B.L. (1999). Influence of periodontal infections of systemic health. *Periodontology 2000* 21: 197.

68 Mealey, B.L. and Klokkevold, P.R. (2006). Periodontal medicine: impact of periodontal infection on systemic health. In: *Carranza's Clinical Periodontology* (eds. F.A. Carranza, M.G. Newman, H.H. Takei and P.R. Klokkevold), 312–329. St. Louis, MO: WB Saunders.

69 Broom, D.M. (2006). Behaviour and welfare in relation to pathology. *Appl. Anim. Behav. Sci.* 97: 73–83.

70 Biondi, M. and Zannino, L.G. (1997). Psychological stress, neuroimmunomodulation, and susceptibility to infectious diseases in animals and man: a review. *Psychother. Psychosom.* 66 (1): 3–26.

71 Karin, M., Lawrence, T., and Nizet, V. (2006). Innate immunity gone awry: linking microbial infections to chronic inflammation and cancer. *Cell* 124 (4): 823–835.

72 Kiank, C., Holtfreter, B., Starke, A. et al. (2006). Stress susceptibility predicts the severity of immune depression and the failure to combat bacterial infections in chronically stressed mice. *Brain Behav. Immun.* 20 (4): 359–368.

73 Rawlinson, J.E., Goldstein, R.E., Reiter, A.M. et al. (2011). Association of periodontal disease with systemic health indices in dogs and the systemic response to treatment of periodontal disease. *J. Am. Vet. Med. Assoc.* 238: 601–609.

74 Nemec, A., Verstraete, F.J., Jerin, A. et al. (2013). Periodontal disease, periodontal treatment and systemic nitric oxide in dogs. *Res. Vet. Sci.* 94: 542–544.

75 Hudson, J.T., Slater, M.R., Taylor, L. et al. (2004). Assessing repeatability and validity of a visual analogue scale questionnaire for use in assessing pain and lameness in dogs. *Am. J. Vet. Res.* 65: 1634–1643.

76 Holton, L., Pawson, P., Nolan, A. et al. (2001). Development of a behaviour-based scale to measure acute pain in dogs. *Vet. Rec.* 148: 525–531.

77 Merola, I. and Mills, D.S. (2016). Behavioural signs of pain in cats: an expert consensus. *PLoS One* 1: e0150040.

78 Furman, R.B. and Niemiec, B.A. (2013). Salivation. In: *Canine and Feline Gastroenterology* (eds. R.J. Washabau and M.J. Day), 162–166. St. Louis, MO: Elsevier.

79 Rusbridge, C. and Heath, S. (2015). Feline orofascial pain syndrome. In: *Feline Behavioural Health and Welfare* (eds. I. Rodan and S. Heath), 213–226. St. Louis, MO: Elsevier.

80 Deforge, D.H. (2009). Identifying and treating oral pain. www.veterinarypracticenews.com/identifying-and-treating-oral-pain (accessed 18 June 2020).

81 (a) Watanabe, R., Doodnaught, G., Proulx, C. et al. (2019). A multidisciplinary study of pain in cats undergoing dental extractions: a prospective, blinded, clinical trial. *PLoS One* 14 (3): e0213195. (b) Hielm-Björkman, A.K., Kuusela, E., Liman, A. et al. (2003). Evaluation of methods for assessment of pain associated with chronic osteoarthritis in dogs. *J. Am. Vet. Med. Assoc.* 222 (11): 1552–1558. 10.2460/javma.2003.222.1552.

82 (a) McElhenny, J. (2005). Taking away the pain. In: *Veterinary Medicine: A Century of Change*, 61–64. WSAVA; (b) McMillan, F.D. (2000, 2000). Quality of life in animals. *J Am Vet Med Assoc* 216: 1904–1910.

83 Niemiec, B.A., Jawor, J., Nemec, A. et al. (2020). World Small Animal Veterinary Association Global Dental Guidelines (full). *JSAP* Volume 61 Issue 7. https://onlinelibrary.wiley.com/doi/10.1111/jsap.13132.

84 Lue, T.W., Pantenburg, D.P., and Crawford, P.M. (2008). Impact of the owner-pet and client-veterinary bond on the care that pets receive. *J. Am. Vet. Med. Assoc.* 232: 531–536.

85 Mariti, C., Pierantoni, L., Sighieri, C. et al. (2017). Guardians' perceptions of dogs' welfare and behaviors related to visiting the veterinary clinic. *J. Appl. Welf. Sci.* 20: 24–33.

86 Knesl, O., Hart, B.L., Fine, A.H. et al. (2016). Opportunities for incorporating the human-animal bond in companion animal practice. *J. Am. Vet. Med. Assoc.* 249 (1): 42–44.

87 Mellor, D. (2016). Updating animal welfare thinking: moving beyond the "five freedoms" towards "a life worth living". *Animals* 6 (3): 21. https://doi.org/10.3390/ani6030021.

88 Doring, D., Roscher, A., Scheipl, F. et al. (2009). Fear related behavior of dogs in veterinary practice. *Vet. J.* 182: 38–43.

89 Gilbert-Gregory, S., Proudfoot, K., Stull, J.W. et al. (2016). Validation of an anxiety tool to assess stress in hospitalized dogs. In: *Proceedings of the Veterinary Behavior Symposium*, San Antonio, 27–28. American College of Veterinary Behaviorists.

90 Edwards, P.T., Smith, B.P., McArthur, M.L. et al. (2019). Fearful Fido: investigating dog experience in the veterinary context in an effort to reduce distress. *Appl. Anim. Behav. Sci.* 213: 14–25.

91 Hekman, J., Karas, A.Z., and Sharp, C.R. (2014). Psychogenic stress in hospitalized dogs; cross species comparisons, implications for health care, and the challenges of evaluation. *Animals* 4: 331–347.

92 Yin, S. (2009). *Low Stress Handling, Restraint and Behavior Modification in Dogs and Cats*. CattleDog Publishing.

93 Herron, M.E. and Shreyer, T. (2014). The pet friendly practice: a guide for practitioners. *Vet. Clin. North Am. Small Anim. Pract.* 44: 451–481.

94 Dreschel, N.A. (2009). Anxiety, fear, disease and lifespan in domestic dogs. *J. Vet. Behav.* 4: 249–250.

95 Hughes, J. (2008). Anaesthesia for the geriatric dog and cat. *Ir. Vet. J.* 61 (6): 380–387.

96 Lloyd, J.K.F. (2017). Minimising stress for patients in the veterinary hospital: why it is important and what can be done about it. *Vet. Sci.* 4 (2): 22.

97 Fields, H.L., Basbaum, A.I., and Heinricher, M.M. (2006). Central nervous system mechanisms of pain modulation. In: *Wall and Melzack's Textbook of Pain*, 5e (eds. S. McMahon and M. Koltzenburg), 130–135. China: Elsevier.

98 Beckman, B. (2013). Patient management for periodontal therapy. In: *Veterinary Periodontology* (ed. B.A. Niemiec), 305–312. Ames: Wiley Blackwell.

99 Landsberg, G.M., Hunthausen, W.L., and Ackerman, L. (2013). *Behavioural Problems of the Dog and Cat*, 3e. Elsevier.

100 Rodan, I., Sundahl, E., Carney, H. et al. (2011). AAFP and ISFM feline-friendly handling guidelines. *J. Feline Med. Surg.* 13: 364–375.

101 Yin, S. (2009). *Low Stress Handling, Restraint and Behavior Modification of Dogs and Cats: Techniques for Patients Who Love their Visits*. Davis, CA, USA: CattleDog Publishing.

102 Siracusa, C., Manteca, X., Cuenca, R. et al. (2010). Effect of a synthetic appeasing pheromone on behavioral, neuroendocrine, immune, and acute-phase perioperative stress responses in dogs. *J. Am. Vet. Med. Assoc.* 237: 673–681.

103 Amat, M., Le Brech, S., Garcia-Marato, C. et al. (2018). Preventing travel anxiety using dexmedetomidine hydrochloride oromucosal gel. In: *Proceedings of 11th International Veterinary Behaviour Meeting* (ed. S. Denenberg), 20–21. Oxfordshire UK: CABI.

104 Rodan, I., Sundahl, E., Carney, H. et al. (2011). AAFP and ISFM feline-friendly handling guidelines. *J. Feline Med. Surg.* 13: 364–375.

105 Gilbert, C., Mikaelsson, A., and Gilbert, S. (2018). Enhancing dogs' welfare during a veterinary consultation; impact of environmental factors and positive interactions before the consultation.

In: *Proceedings of the 1st Annual Meeting of the European Congress of Behavioral Medicine and Animal Welfare, Berlin*, 254–255.

106 Korpivaara, M., Huhtinen, M., Aspergren, J. et al. (2018). Dexemedetomidine oromucosal gel for alleviation of fear and anxiety in dogs during minor veterinary or husbandry procedures. In: *Proceedings of 11th International Veterinary Behaviour Meeting* (ed. S. Denenberg), 22–23. Oxfordshire, UK: CABI.

107 Lansberg, G., Hunthausen, W., and Ackerman, L. (2013). Prevention: the best medicine. In: *Behaviour Problems of the Dog & Cat*, 39–64. Saunders Elsevier.

108 Todd, Z. (2018). Review. Barriers to the adoption of humane dog training methods. *J. Vet. Behav.* 25: 28–34.

109 Ziv, G. (2017). The effects of using aversive training methods in dogs: a review. *J. Vet. Behav.* 19: 50–60.

110 Hernander L. (2008). Factors Influencing Dogs' Stress Level in the Waiting Room at a Veterinary Clinic. Student Report. Swedish University of Agricultural Sciences, Department of Animal Environment and Health, Ethology and Animal Welfare Programme. https://stud.epsilon.slu.se/10787/1/hernander_l_170913.pdf (accessed 11 August 2020).

111 Mariti, C., Raspanti, E., Zilocchi, M. et al. (2015). The assessment of dog welfare in the waiting room of a veterinary clinic. *Anim. Welfare* 24: 299–305.

112 Hekman, J.P., Karas, A.Z., and Dreschel, N.A. (2012). Salivary cortisol concentrations and behavior in a population of healthy dogs hospitalized for elective procedures. *Appl. Anim. Behav. Sci.* 141: 149–157.

113 Bragg, R.F., Bennett, J.S., Cummings, A. et al. (2015). Evaluations of the effects of hospital stress on physiologic variables in dogs. *J. Am. Vet. Med. Assoc.* 246: 212–215.

114 Engler, W. and Bain, M. (2017). Effect of different types of classical music played at a veterinary hospital on dog behavior and owner satisfaction. *J. Am. Vet. Med. Assoc.* 251: 195–200.

115 Benson, G.J., Grubb, T.L., Neff-Davis, C. et al. (2000). Perioperative stress response in the dog; effect of pre-emptive administration of medetomidine. *Vet. Surg.* 29: 85–89.

116 Savvas, I., Rallis, T., and Raptopoulos, D. (2009). The effect of pre-anesthetic fasting time and type of food on gastric content volume and acidity in dogs. *Vet. Anaesth. Analg.* 36: 539–546.

117 Westlund, K. (2015). To feed or not to feed: counterconditioning in the veterinary clinic. *J. Vet. Behav.* 10: 433–437.

118 Savvas, I., Raptopoulos, D., and Rallis, T. (2016). A "light meal" three hours pre-operatively decreases the incidence of gastro-esophageal reflux in dogs. *J. Am. Anim. Hosp. Assoc.* https://doi.org/10.5326/JAAHA-MS-639.

119 Tunnell, J.C. and Harrel, S.K. (2017). Minimally invasive surgery in periodontal regeneration: a review of the literature. *Compend. Contin. Educ. Dent.* 38 (4): e13–e16. Review.

120 Cortellini, P. and Tonetti, M.S. (2007). A minimally invasive surgical technique with an enamel matrix derivative in the regenerative treatment of intra-bony defects: a novel approach to limit morbidity. *J. Clin. Periodontol.* 34 (1): 87–93.

121 Kumar, A., Yadav, N., Singh, S., and Chauhan, N. (2016). Minimally invasive (endoscopic-computer assisted) surgery: technique and review. *Ann. Maxillofac. Surg.* 6 (2): 159–164.

122 Niemiec, B.A. (2012). *Dental Extractions Made Easier*. Tustin: Practical Veterinary Publishing.

123 Stiles, J., Weil, A.B., and Packer, R.A. (2012). Post-anesthetic cortical blindness in cats: twenty cases. *Vet. J.* 193 (2): 367–373.

124 de Miguel Garcia, C., Whiting, M., and Alibhai, H. (2013). Cerebral hypoxia in a cat following pharyngoscopy involving use of a mouth gag. *Vet. Anaesth. Analg.* 40 (1): 106–108.

125 Niemiec, B.A. (2013). The complete dental cleaning. In: *Veterinary Periodontology* (ed. B.A. Niemiec), 129–153. Ames: Wiley Blackwell.

126 Bellows, J. (2004). Periodontal equipment, materials, and techniques. In: *Small Animal Dental Equipment, Materials, and Techniques, a Primer*, 115–173. Blackwell.

127 Holmstrom, S.E., Frost, P., and Eisner, E.R. (2002). Dental prophylaxis and periodontal disease stages. In: *Veterinary Dental Techniques*, 3e, 175–232. Philadelphia, PA: Saunders.

128 Carranza, F.A. and Takei, H.H. (2006). Clinical diagnosis. In: *Carranza's Clinical Periodontology* (eds. F.A. Carranza, M.G. Newman, H.H. Takei and P.R. Klokkevold), 540–560. St. Louis, MO: WB Saunders.

129 Niemiec, B.A. (2011). The importance of dental radiology. *Eur. J. Comp. Anim. Pract.* 20 (3): 219–229.

130 Tsugawa, A.J. and Verstraete, F.J. (2000). How to obtain and interpret periodontal radiographs in dogs. *Clin. Tech. Small Anim. Pract.* 15 (4): 204–210.

131 Verstraete, F.J., Kass, P.H., and Terpak, C.H. (1998). Diagnostic value of full-mouth radiography in cats. *Am. J. Vet. Res.* 59 (6): 692–695.

132 Niemiec, B.A. (2008). Case based dental radiology. *Top. Companion Anim. Med.* 24 (1): 4–19.

133 Colmery, B. (2005). The gold standard of veterinary oral health care, in (ed. S.E. Holmstrolm). *Vet. Clin. North Am.* 35 (4): 781–787.

134 Niemiec, B.A. (2003). Professional teeth cleaning. *J. Vet. Dent.* 20 (3): 175–180.

135 Duffy, D.L., Hsu, Y., and Serpell, J.A. (2008). Breed differences in canine aggression. *Appl. Anim. Behav. Sci.* 114: 441–460.

4

Conditions Commonly Seen in Brachycephalic Breeds

Brook A. Niemiec

Veterinary Dental Specialties and Oral Surgery, San Diego, CA, USA

4.1 Class III Malocclusions

A malocclusion was classically defined as any bite which is abnormal for the breed. Therefore, by this definition, class III malocclusions were actually considered normal in brachycephalic breeds (termed a class 0, type III malocclusion) [1, 2], However, the American Veterinary Dental College and the WSAVA dental guidelines committee defines a malocclusion as occurring whenever a tooth or teeth are not able to fit comfortably when the mouth is closed [3, 4]. Therefore, if *any* occlusal trauma is present, appropriate therapy should be recommended and expediently performed [5]. Occasionally, no occlusal trauma will occur with a class III malocclusion, thus it is purely cosmetic and no therapy is necessary (Figure 4.1). However, patients with malocclusions may be more prone to periodontal disease [6, 7]. This is especially true if the teeth are visible outside of the mouth (see Figure 4.1a), which will lead to decreased salivary action, which has been shown to increase periodontal disease [8].

Class III malocclusions can create several different types of damage to the teeth and oral soft tissues [1, 5, 9].

a) Soft tissue trauma to the mandibular gingiva from the maxillary incisors (Figure 4.2). This often occurs distal to the incisors and may create significant gingival damage. In addition, contact may occur in the gingival sulcus and create periodontal inflammation and disease. Unfortunately, this painful condition is rarely diagnosed and often considered "normal". Treatment consists of extraction or coronal reduction and either bonded sealant or endodontic therapy of the offending teeth [1, 10, 11].

b) Tooth-to-tooth contact of the maxillary third incisors and mandibular canines [12]. Depending on the severity of the discrepancy, this can result in significant attrition to the mandibular canines, and may contribute to fracture of the tooth (Figure 4.3). In these cases, extraction or crown reduction and endodontic therapy of the maxillary third incisors will alleviate the trauma. The canine is best treated with a cast metal crown, as it is the only therapy that will increase the strength of the tooth of any appreciable level (Figure 4.4). The other option for the canine is a composite restoration, but this provides minimal strength.

Breed Predispositions to Dental and Oral Disease in Dogs, First Edition. Edited by Brook A. Niemiec.
© 2021 John Wiley & Sons, Inc. Published 2021 by John Wiley & Sons, Inc.

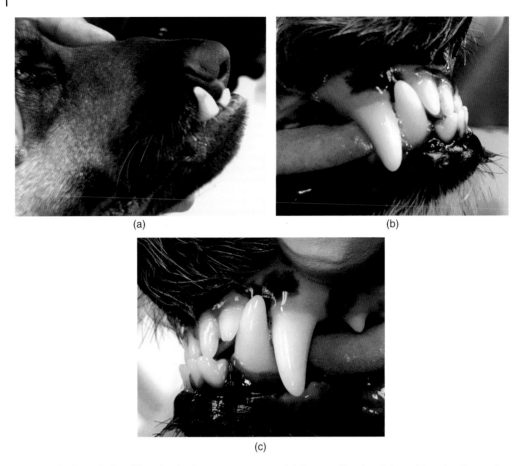

Figure 4.1 Not all class III malocclusions create trauma. (a) German Shepherd dog with a significant class III malocclusion. The jaws are far enough off to not be creating any trauma. No therapy is necessary. (b & c) Shih Tzu with a mild class III malocclusion (reverse scissors) bite from the right (b) and left (c) side. The teeth rest comfortably in the mouth. This is a cosmetic situation only and no therapy is recommended.

c) Traumatic pulpitis of the mandibular canine, which may result in endodontic disease and possibly abscessation [12, 13]. This will be evidenced by intrinsic staining (discoloration) of the affected tooth (Figure 4.5). If this occurs, endodontic therapy or extraction is necessary [14].

d) Upper lip trauma and secondary ulceration [11]. This situation may be treated by extraction or coronal amputation and endodontic therapy of the mandibular canines.

e) Incorrect alignment of the maxillary and mandibular premolars. This may cause tooth-to-tooth trauma resulting in attrition (wear) and/or traumatic pulpitis [1, 13]. This may be treated by extraction or endodontic therapy [14].

f) Mild class III malocclusions (level bites) may create incisor on incisor contact, leading to (potentially significant) attrition (Figure 4.6). While this is rare in brachycephalic breeds as the discrepancy is generally more severe, if diagnosed, treatment is necessary. If the trauma is mild, coronal reeducation and bonded sealants can be sufficient. In severe cases, extraction of the teeth on one arcade should be considered.

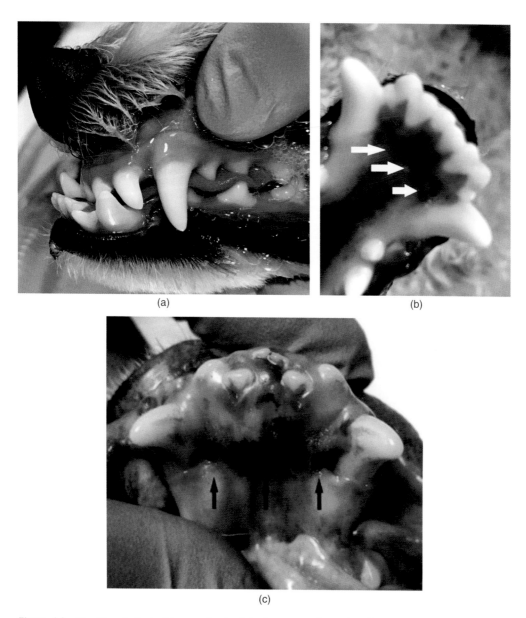

(a)

(b)

(c)

Figure 4.2 Significant gingival trauma (and pain) often occurs from class III malocclusions, even though it is rarely diagnosed. (a) A young canine patient with a significant class III malocclusion with the mandibular canines rostral to the third incisors. The trauma is not easily evident on the conscious exam. (b) Intraoral dental picture of the patient in (a) showing gingival trauma from the maxillary first and second incisors (white arrows). (c) Intraoral dental picture of a Boxer showing gingival trauma from the maxillary first and second incisors (black arrows). Image courtesy of Rob Yelland and previously published in "Veterinary Orthodontics". Source: Used with permission from Practical Veterinary Publishing.

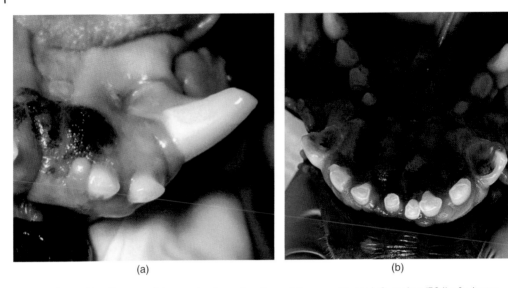

(a)   (b)

Figure 4.3 (a) Significant attrition on the lingual surface of the mandibular left canine (304) of a boxer from contact with the ipsilateral third incisor (203). This is not only painful, but also significantly weakens the tooth and predisposes it to fracture. There is also gingival recession in the area due to the occlusal trauma. (b) Intraoral dental picture showing the mandibular canines (304 and 404) with severe attrition from the maxillary third incisors. The weakening eventually resulted in fracture of the teeth and secondary endodontic infection.

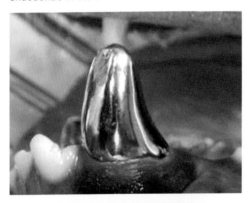

Figure 4.4 A cast metal titanium alloy crown applied to the tooth in Figure 4.3. This extends below the weakened area on the lingual aspect and will help prevent fracture of the tooth.

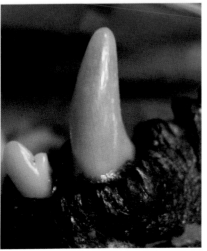

Figure 4.5 An intrinsically stained (discolored) left mandibular canine (304) in a dog with occlusal trauma. This tooth is non-vital and requires root canal therapy or extraction.

Figure 4.6 A mild class III malocclusion (level bite) which has created incisor on incisor contact and secondary attrition to the teeth. This also increases the chance of tooth fracture.

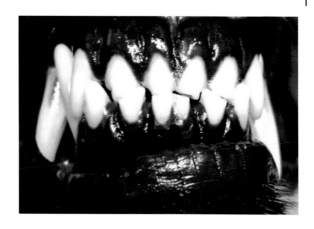

4.1.1 Brachycephalic Syndrome

This is a combination of stenotic nares, elongated soft palate, and everted saccules. These conditions can create significant breathing issues for the patient; if this is the case, they should be surgically corrected. This will improve the pet's ventilation, but will not make it normal. (See separate chapters on this condition.)

References

1 Niemiec, B.A. (2010). *Pathology in the Pediatric Patient* (ed. B.A. Niemiec), 89–126. London: Manson.

2 Niemiec, B.A. (2013). Deciduous malocclusions. In: *Veterinary Orthodontics* (ed. B.A. Niemiec), 17–21. Tustin: Practical Veterinary Publishing.

3 American Veterinary Dental College and the WSAVA Dental Guidelines Committee (2019). Malocclusion. http://AVDC.org/nomenclature (accessed 19 June 2020).

4 World Small Animal Veterinary Association (2019). Malocclusion. http://WSAVA.org (accessed 19 June 2020).

5 Lobprise, H.B. (2019). Occlusion and Othodontics. In: *Wiggs' Veterinary Dentistry Principals and Practice*, 2e (eds. H.B. Lobprise and J.R. Dodd), 411–437. Hoboken: Wiley Blackwell.

6 Abu Alhaija, E.S. and Al-Wahadni, A.M. (2006). Relationship between tooth irregularity and periodontal disease in children with regular dental visits. *J. Clin. Pediatr. Dent.* 30 (4): 296–298.

7 Feng, X., Oba, T., Oba, Y., and Moriyama, K. (2005). An interdisciplinary approach for improved functional and esthetic results in a periodontally compromised adult patient. *Angle Orthod.* 25 (6): 1061–1070.

8 Gupta, O.P., Blechman, H., and Stahl, S.S. (1960). The effects of desalivation on periodontal tissues of the Syrian hamster. *Oral Surg. Oral Med. Oral Pathol.* 13: 470–481.

9 Yelland, R. (2013). Class III malocclusions. In: *Veterinary Orthodontics* (ed. B.A. Niemiec), 110–115. Tustin: Practical Veterinary Publishing.

10 Wiggs, R.B. and Lobprise, H.B. (1997). *Veterinary Dentistry, Principles and Practice*. Philadelphia: Lippincott-Raven.

11 Harvey, C.E. and Emily, P.P. (1993). *Small Animal Dentistry*. St. Louis: Mosby.

12 Hale, F.A. (2005). Juvenile veterinary dentistry. *Vet. Clin. Small Anim.* (35, 4): 789–817.

13 Brine, E.J. (1999). Endodontic disease of the mandibular first molar tooth secondary to caudal cross bite in a young Shetland sheepdog. *J. Vet. Dent.* 16 (1): 15–18.

14 DuPont, G.G. (2010). Problems with the dental hard tissues. In: *Small Animal Dental, Oral and Maxillofacial Disease, a Color Handbook* (ed. B.A. Niemiec), 127–157. London: Manson.

5

Brachycephalic Airway Disease

Sean W. Aiken

Veterinary Specialty Hospital, San Diego, CA, USA

Brachycephalic airway syndrome (BAS), also known as brachycephalic obstructive airway syndrome (BOAS) and brachycephalic airway obstruction syndrome (BAOS), is a condition associated with selective breeding that results in decreased maxillary length without a concurrent decrease in the soft tissue volume in the nasal cavity and pharyngeal region. This syndrome gives rise to primary anatomic abnormalities of the upper airway including stenotic nares, elongated soft palate, hypoplastic trachea, and aberrant nasopharyngeal turbinates. These anatomic abnormalities result in chronic partial upper airway obstruction and increased upper airway resistance, which can result in secondary complications that may include inflammation, mucosal, and cartilage changes leading to everted laryngeal saccules, laryngeal collapse, pharyngeal collapse, and eversion of the tonsils [1–4]. Chronic upper airway obstruction can also result in myofiber degeneration and denervation of the palatine and hyoepiglotticus muscles, which can worsen upper airway collapse, and can lead to edematous and redundant mucosa, and even epiglottic retroversion. These progressive changes can lead to a worsening of the BAOS and life-threatening upper respiratory compromise [5–7]. Nasopharyngeal sialoceles have been reported as a rare consequence of chronic stresses to the mucosa and salivary glands within the nasopharynx in brachycephalic dogs [8].

Common brachycephalic breeds include Pugs, English bulldogs, French bulldogs, Boston terriers, Pekingese, Maltese, Shih Tzus, boxers, Cavalier King Charles spaniels, Yorkshire terriers, miniature pinschers, and Chihuahuas [9] to name a few. As the popularity of brachycephalic breeds has increased in recent years, the familiarity of the specific conditions and treatment options for BAOS has become an important aspect of veterinary practice [10, 11]. The diagnosis of BAOS is based on history, physical examination findings, sedated pharyngeal/laryngeal examination, endoscopy, and diagnostic imaging. The primary causes of BAOS and the secondary effects of chronic increased airway resistance need to be differentiated from other conditions that can result in respiratory obstruction, including laryngeal paralysis, collapsing trachea, neoplasia that results in fixed or dynamic obstructions, and trauma.

Epiglottic retroversion is a condition where there is spontaneous epiglottic retroflexion during inspiration causing obstruction of the rima glottidis (laryngeal opening) and must be ruled out as a cause of progressive upper airway obstruction. This condition can be seen in brachiocephalic dogs as well as other breeds and can be a cause of progressive, intermittent severe upper airway obstruction in typically older to middle-aged dogs [7]. The cause of epiglottic retroversion is

Breed Predispositions to Dental and Oral Disease in Dogs, First Edition. Edited by Brook A. Niemiec.
© 2021 John Wiley & Sons, Inc. Published 2021 by John Wiley & Sons, Inc.

unknown, but thought to be secondary to hyoepiglotticus muscle dysfunction due to myopathy or neuropathy from hypoglossal nerve dysfunction. Epiglottic cartilage degeneration or fracture has been a cause of epiglottic retroversion in people [12]. Epiglottic retroversion is diagnosed by upper airway fluoroscopy and sedated laryngeal examination, and must be included in the differential diagnosis of dogs with intermittent severe or progressive upper airway obstruction.

5.1 History and Clinical Signs

The presenting clinical signs and their severity in dogs with BAOS varies dramatically, but can include stridor, inspiratory dyspnea, hyperthermia, sleep apnea, and in severe cases, syncope and collapse [1]. Age of presentation is wide-ranging, from less than six months of age to middle age, and rarely initial diagnosis may occur in older dogs. With time, more negative pressure is required to breathe, resulting in collapse of the soft tissues of the pharyngeal region; thereby the clinical signs typically worsen with age.

Increased environmental temperature, especially during the warm summer months, tends to exacerbate clinical respiratory signs, leading to limitations in exercise tolerance and lengthening of exercise recovery time [13, 14]. Obesity has been shown to negatively affect both respiratory function and heat tolerance in brachycephalic dogs, compared with dogs with normal airway confirmation [13].

Clinical signs may not be specific to the upper airway system, as affected dogs may also exhibit gastrointestinal signs including salivation, regurgitation, and vomiting [14–16]. Gastrointestinal signs may have breed-specific tendencies, for instance affected French bulldogs tend to have more eating/digestive problems than pugs [14, 16]. Hiatal hernias are also common in dogs presenting with BAOS and gastrointestinal signs [4]. Correction of the upper airway obstruction in brachycephalic dogs can alleviate many of the gastrointestinal signs [17]. If the gastrointestinal signs do not improve after correction for BAS, then additional testing may need to be performed to address them [15].

The severity of the clinical signs will vary significantly depending on the animal's age, severity of the primary anatomic changes, and progression of the secondary airway and gastrointestinal changes.

5.2 Physical Examination

Physical examination, both at rest and with activity, will help determine the severity of the upper airway obstruction. Observation of breathing patterns to assess for inspiratory and/or expiratory stertor will help determine if the patient is suffering from upper or lower airway disease (or fixed obstruction). Owner provided videos of specific episodes can help identify situational causes and severity of the obstructive episodes. Auscultation of the lungs in patients with BAOS will often be complicated by referred upper airway noise, which often limits evaluation of lung sounds. Auscultation of the laryngeal region and trachea can aid in identifying the region of greatest turbulent flow and therefore greatest obstruction and should be performed at rest as well as after mild exercise [18].

Stenotic nares can be noted on conscious physical examination and can be classified as mild, moderate, or severe (Figure 5.1). Clinical significance of the stenotic nares is confirmed through observation of medial deviation of the wing of the nostril (*ala nasi*) with inspiration, which results in collapse and obstruction of the nasal opening [19].

Figure 5.1 Moderately stenotic nares.

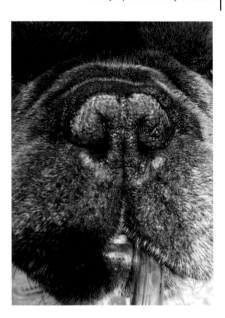

5.3 Pharyngeal/Laryngeal Examination

Laryngeal/pharyngeal examination is required to diagnose the pharyngeal and laryngeal components of BAOS. Examination is performed under a light plane of anesthesia, without placement of an endotracheal tube. If tractable, the patient is ideally preoxygenated with a mask and oxygen supplementation should be provided throughout the procedure with flow by. Anesthesia can be induced with propofol (3 mg kg^{-1}, IV), with additional boluses (0.75 mg kg^{-1}, IV) administered as needed [20]. Oral cavity visualization is maintained using a gentle mouth gag or by suspension of the maxilla and retraction of the mandible through the placement of gauze loops around the upper and lower canine teeth. A laryngoscope blade may be used to displace the tongue ventrally to assess the relative location of the soft palate and the epiglottis when the soft tissues are in a natural position. Use caution as placing forward traction on the tongue will alter the position of the larynx and epiglottis, thereby displacing and distorting the natural landmarks. An elongated palate is diagnosed when the soft palate extends over the tip of the epiglottis by 2–3 mm or more (Figure 5.2).

The soft palate can then be elevated using a tongue depressor, or similar instrument, and the larynx evaluated for evidence of normal abduction of the arytenoid cartilage to rule out laryngeal paralysis and to assess for signs of laryngeal collapse. The ideal time to assess laryngeal function is within two to five minutes after anesthetic induction [20]. Doxapram (Dopram 2.2 mg kg^{-1}, IV) can be used to stimulate respiration to better assess laryngeal function and dynamic effects of breathing during the laryngeal examination [20].

The three recognized stages of laryngeal collapse progress in severity from the ventral to dorsal aspect of the larynx. Stage 1 is eversion of the laryngeal saccules, evidenced by small outpouchings of laryngeal mucosa just rostral to the vocal folds (Figure 5.3). They typically are clear to white in color but can be red and edematous in dogs with clinically severe obstruction. Stage 2 laryngeal collapse is defined as the collapsing of the cuneiform process of the arytenoid cartilage into the laryngeal lumen. Stage 3 is identified by the collapsing of the corniculate process toward midline, resulting in the occlusion of the rima glottidis [21]. The presence of redundant and/or edematous

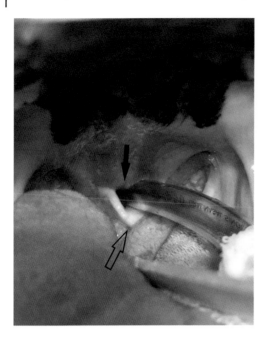

Figure 5.2 Elongated soft palate. Note the edge of the soft palate (solid arrow) is caudal the edge of the epiglottis (open arrow).

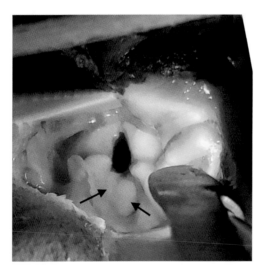

Figure 5.3 Eversion of the laryngeal saccules (black arrows).

mucosa and enlarged and edematous tonsils should be evaluated and documented [6]. In patients with epiglottic retroversion, the epiglottis is noted to intermittently move caudally during inspiration and can result in complete obstruction of the rima glottidis (Figure 5.4). The epiglottis in these cases can appear flattened, and if recent the cause of obstruction may appear erythematous and edematous (Figure 5.5) [7]. After the pharyngeal/laryngeal examination is complete, the patient can be intubated and maintained on inhalant anesthesia if additional diagnostics and/or procedures are planned.

Figure 5.4 Epiglottic retroversion. The epiglottis (white star) moves caudally with inspiration and occludes the rima glottidis. Note the epiglottis is trapped caudal to the soft palate (white arrows).

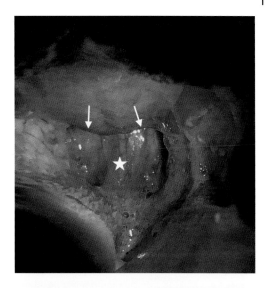

Figure 5.5 An inflamed dorsal surface of the epiglottis after reduction of epiglottic retroversion.

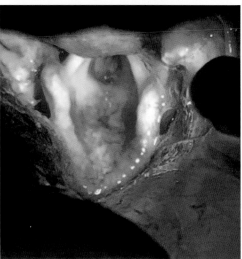

5.4 Diagnostic Imaging

Thoracic radiographs should be performed to assess for concurrent conditions such as hypoplastic trachea, pneumonia, hiatal hernia (Figure 5.6), and cardiovascular abnormalities (heart enlargement, pulmonary edema). The tracheal diameter (TD) at the thoracic inlet (TI) to the thoracic inlet diameter ratio (TD:TI) of less than 0.2 in most breeds is consistent with hypoplastic trachea (Figure 5.6). Since English bulldogs have a relatively narrow trachea normal in the breed, a TD:TI ratio of less than 0.12 is consistent with hypoplastic trachea in this breed [22, 23].

Computed tomography (CT) of the skull and nasal cavities may be performed to evaluate the obstructing soft tissue components of BAOS, including soft palate dimensions (thickness and

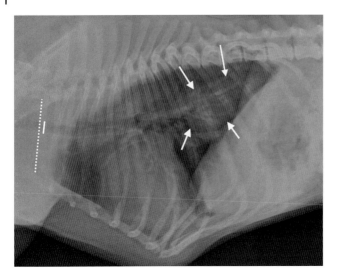

Figure 5.6 Lateral thoracic radiographic image of a one-year-old French bulldog presenting for BAOS surgery. Note the soft issue mass effect in the caudal thorax (white arrows) consistent with a hiatal hernia. A tracheal diameter (TD) (solid white line) to thoracic inlet (TI) (white dotted line) ratio (TD:TI) is used to evaluate for a hypoplastic trachea.

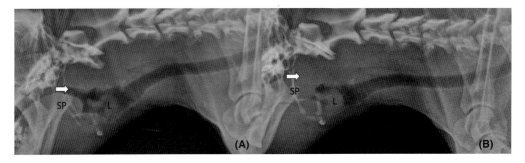

Figure 5.7 (A) During expiration, the nasopharynx is open, having a distinct air column (arrow). (B) During inspiration, the nasopharynx collapses, resulting in attenuation of the nasopharyngeal air column (arrow). On both images, there is thickening of the soft palate and soft tissue opacification of the larynx suggesting eversion of the laryngeal saccules. (SP = soft palate; L = larynx). Source: Images courtesy of Rachael Pollard DVM, Ph.D., DACVR. University of California, Davis.

length), the presence of abnormal or aberrant nasopharyngeal turbinates (rostral and caudal), deviation of the septum and tracheal dimensions [24–27]. It is important to consider that a CT evaluation is static in nature, while BAOS is a dynamic soft tissue condition. CT scan evaluation of the pharyngeal diameter and soft tissue structures can be affected by intubation during anesthesia [26].

Videofluoroscopy can be used to assess the soft tissue components of patients with BAOS and has the advantage of visualization of the dynamic obstructing conditions during various phases of respiration. It has the advantage of radiographic assessment of the dynamic changes in the pharynx, larynx, and trachea and can be very useful in cases of pharyngeal collapse (Figure 5.7) and epiglottic retroversion (Figure 5.8) [2, 7]. This is typically performed in the awake or lightly sedated patient.

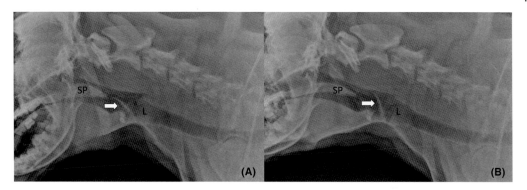

Figure 5.8 (A) During expiration, the epiglottis (arrow) is positioned so that the rima glottidis is unobstructed. (B) During inspiration, the epiglottis is retroflexed (arrow) causing partial obstruction of the rima glottidis. On both images, there is caudal retraction of the hyoid apparatus and larynx consistent with upper airway obstruction. (SP = soft palate; L = larynx). Source: Images courtesy of Rachael Pollard DVM, Ph.D., DACVR. University of California, Davis.

Videoendoscopy is beneficial for direct evaluation of the entire nasopharynx, nasal cavity, larynx, as well as the upper and lower airways. Nasopharyngeal turbinates can be assessed, while evaluating the degree and extent of laryngeal, tracheal, and bronchial collapse [28, 29]. This modality can also complement CT scan findings of intranasal and nasopharyngeal abnormalities and may be of value in planning surgery in dogs affected with BAOS [8, 30]. Finally, Videoendoscopy can also be used to evaluate the upper gastrointestinal tract in dogs with BAOS that present for regurgitation and vomiting.

5.5 Diagnostic Testing

Brachycephalic breeds suffer from chronic hypoxia (lower PaO_2), hypercapnia (higher $PaCO_2$), higher red blood cell volumes (higher packed cell volume [PCV]) and hypertension compared to nonbrachycephalic dogs [31]. Current bloodwork including a complete blood count and serum biochemistry panel should be performed as a baseline prior to anesthesia. Pulse oximetry and/or arterial blood gasses can be used to assess for hypoxemia. Although pulse oximetry levels are often lower in brachycephalic breeds than mesocephalic dogs, hypoxemia should never be considered normal, and treatment should be initiated if hypoxemia is diagnosed [32]. Resting blood pressure measurements should be performed to diagnose preexisting hypertension, which should be addressed prior to anesthesia.

5.6 Measuring Airflow Resistance

Recently there have been attempts to objectify measurements of airflow resistance in dogs. There are several options that may be available in the future, including CT scan and computational fluid dynamics models of nasal airflow resistance [33], as well as whole-body barometric plethysmography. The latter is a non-invasive technique that can measure respiratory function. The dog is placed in a chamber, and changes in pressure within the chamber can be used to extrapolate tidal volume and respiratory function. The advantages are that the patient can be measured awake, at rest, and while sleeping [34, 35]. These tests may be useful for guidance and objective measurements of the severity of the upper airway obstruction as well as evaluation of the effects of surgical procedures.

5.7 Surgical Treatment

Initial treatment of BAOS should be performed when the tissues have matured to a point that they will hold suture, as early as three to six months of age. Although correction of the primary causes of BAOS at an early age to prevent secondary changes from becoming clinical is preferable, older patients will still benefit from surgery [36]. Suction should be available during surgery to remove blood and secretions from the surgery site and to clear the pharynx, nasal cavity, and larynx prior to recovery. Personal magnification (loupes) and a headlamp light source can facilitate the procedure. Access to the caudal pharynx can be challenging in brachycephalic breeds, therefore long surgical instruments including fine/long needle holders, long curved Metzenbaum scissors, and long Debakey forceps, can aid the surgeon in these procedures.

Gastrointestinal signs are common with dogs suffering from BAOS. Surgery on the upper airway as well as the hospital environment can also cause anxiety in our patients which can have a profound impact on potential post-operative complications. Pre-treatment with maropitant ($2\,\mathrm{mg\,kg^{-1}}$ PO q 24 hours), omeprazole ($1\,\mathrm{mg\,kg^{-1}}$ PO q 12–24 hours) [37] and trazodone (3.5–$7\,\mathrm{mg\,kg^{-1}}$) [38] starting the day before surgery is recommended. The patient should be treated with an anti-inflammatory dose of dexamethasone sodium phosphate at $0.01\,\mathrm{mg\,kg^{-1}}$ IV ($0.5\,\mathrm{mg\,kg^{-1}}$ of prednisone equivalent where dexamethasone is six times more potent than prednisone) at the time of anesthetic induction.

5.8 Stenotic Nares

There are several techniques that are successful at permanently widening the nares, including alar amputation, wedge resection, punch alaplasty, and alapexy [39–41]. These techniques are typically aimed at removal of a portion of the wing of the nostril with a #11 blade or a skin biopsy punch to widen the nares, or by permanently fixing the ala nasi in an abducted position. The technique chosen is primarily surgeon preference, but in this author's opinion, different techniques can have a significant effect on the cosmetic outcome. The two common techniques described below should be performed following sterile preparation of the nasal plenum.

5.8.1 Wedge Resection Technique

A triangular-shaped wedge of tissue is removed from the wing of the nostril and extending caudally to include the alar cartilage by inserting a #11 blade at the apex of the wedge, starting at the dorsal extent of the nares, 2 mm lateral to and parallel to the medial edge of the cartilage. The blade is inserted in a caudal direction and extended through the ventral aspect of the wing of the nostril. A second incision is started at the apex and aimed caudally to meet the first incision and directed laterally and ventrally to create and remove a triangular wedge of the lateral nares. The width of the wedge defines the resultant opening of the nares (Figure 5.9). The caudal extent of the incision should include a portion of the alar cartilage to assure there is adequate space for nasal airflow. Hemostasis is achieved with gentle digital pressure or by placing a sterile cotton tipped applicator in the nares to appose the two cut surfaces. The edges of the incision are closed with 4 or more fine

Figure 5.9 Wedge resection rhinoplasty. A wedge-shaped segment of the wing of the nostril, which extends caudally to the alar fold, is removed.

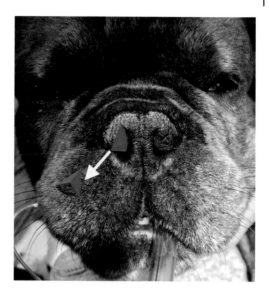

Figure 5.10 Post-operative wedge rhinoplasty. The edges of the incision are closed with fine absorbable suture material in an interrupted pattern. Symmetry of the new nasal opening is achieved by removal of the same amount of tissue from both sides of the wing of the nostril. Swelling at the time of surgery can make determination of symmetry difficult.

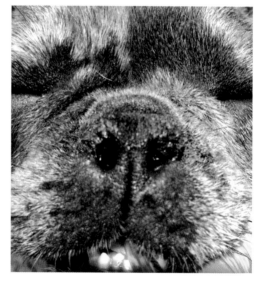

(4–0 or 5–0) absorbable sutures in an interrupted pattern, taking care to suture the ventral portion of the wing of the nostril. The technique is repeated on the opposite wing of the nostril, taking care to remove the same size wedge to assure symmetry of the nares [40] (Figure 5.10).

5.8.2 Punch Alaplasty Technique

An appropriately sized disposable skin biopsy punch (2–6 mm in diameter) is used to remove a cylinder of tissue from the wing of the nostril and alar cartilage. The size of the skin biopsy instrument is chosen such that 2 mm of tissue remains medial and lateral to the resected cylinder of tissue. The caudal end of cylindrical excised piece of tissue is then cut with iris scissors. Additional alar cartilage can be removed as needed with iris scissors (Figure 5.11). Hemostasis is achieved with gentle digital pressure or by placing a sterile cotton tipped applicator in the nares to appose

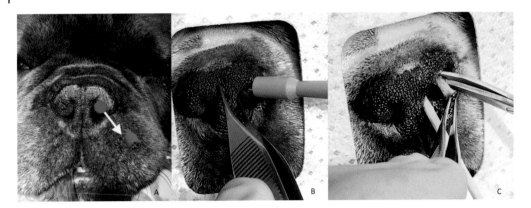

Figure 5.11 Punch alaplasty (A). An appropriately sized sharp skin punch is used to remove a columnar segment of the wing of the nostril (B). The core of tissue must extend caudally to remove any obstructing alar cartilage (C).

the two cut surfaces. The edges of the incision are closed using 3–4 fine (4–0 or 5–0) absorbable sutures in an interrupted pattern [41].

5.9 Elongated Soft Palate

There are several techniques for correction of an elongated soft palate. The technique chosen is mainly the surgeon's preference, but can be influenced by the availability of equipment or the thickness of the soft palate. The patient is positioned in either sternal or dorsal recumbency (surgeon preference) with the mouth held open with tape strips or a mouth gag (Figure 5.12). Gauze sponges are placed in the caudal pharynx to protect the airway while the oral cavity is prepared with a chlorhexidine oral rinse.

5.9.1 Soft Palate Resection (Staphylectomy)

Shortening of the soft palate can be performed with scissors using a cut and sew technique, a carbon dioxide laser, bipolar or monopolar electrocautery or a vessel sealing device (Monnet 2004) [23, 36, 42, 43]. Laser resection of the soft palate has been shown to decrease surgical times [36] but there have been no differences in outcome based on surgical technique used. If a laser is to be used, the endotracheal tube must be protected, and all laser safety precautions strictly adhered to.

The soft palate should be shortened such that the caudal edge of the soft palate just touches the tip of the epiglottis when the tongue is in a neutral position. Another landmark is that the caudal margin of the soft palate should be at the level of the caudal to central aspect of the tonsillar crypt. The ideal length of the soft palate has not been determined; however, excessive resection of the soft palate could result in nasopharyngeal reflux. However, resection of the soft palate to the level of the cranial tonsillar crypt did not result in nasopharyngeal reflux in one study [44]. The caudal margin of the soft palate at the midline is grasped with Allis tissue forceps (Figure 5.13a); alternatively, a traction suture can be placed to retract the soft palate rostrally. With the tongue in a neutral position, the site of soft palate resection is determined. A suture of fine synthetic absorbable suture (4–0 to 5–0) is placed at the lateral margin of the soft palate at the desired resection level

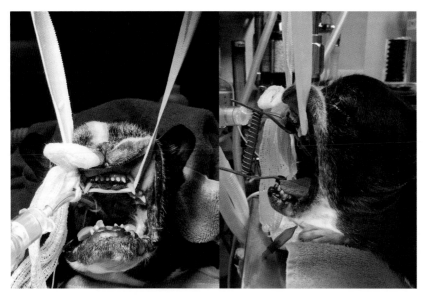

Figure 5.12 Positioning of a dog in sternal recumbency (frontal and lateral views) with the mandible suspended and mouth gag in place.

and tied (Figure 5.13b). The non-needled tail of the suture should be tagged with a hemostat to help with manipulation. The traditional cut and sew technique (author's preference) is then performed by partial transection of full thickness soft palate with long curved Metzenbaum scissors (Figure 5.13c), starting adjacent to your pre-placed lateral suture and extending toward the centerline. Approximately 1/3 of the width of the soft palate is transected at a time, followed by suturing the nasal and oral mucosa with the needle end of the lateral pre-placed suture in a simple continuous pattern. Minimal bleeding is typically encountered and is controlled with pressure from the suture. The cut then sew procedure is continued until the soft palate resection is completed at the desired level (Figure 5.13d). The caudal pharynx is suctioned and the pharyngeal packing is removed.

5.9.2   Folded Flap Palatopasty

While this author does not perform or generally recommend this technique, in patients with an elongated, as well as a thickened soft palate, the folded flap palatoplasty can both shorten and decrease the thickness of the soft palate [45]. The caudal margin of the soft palate is grasped with forceps or traction sutures and folded rostrally along the ventral soft palate until the folded caudal edge of the soft palate is at an appropriate final length for the soft palate, and this site is marked on the ventral (oral) mucosa. This mark is typically 1–2 cm caudal to the palatine processes of the palatine bone [45]. The ventral (oral) mucosa of the soft palate is resected in a trapezoid shape, extending caudally from this site to the caudal edge of the soft palate and laterally to just medial to the tonsillar crypts. The palatine musculature is then resected, leaving the nasopharyngeal mucosa and submucosa of the soft palate. The caudal edge of the soft palate is then folded rostrally to the rostral margin of the resection, and the folded nasopharyngeal soft palate mucosa is sutured to the oral mucosa of the soft palate using fine synthetic absorbable sutures (4–0 to 5–0). The resultant soft palate is shorter and thinner.

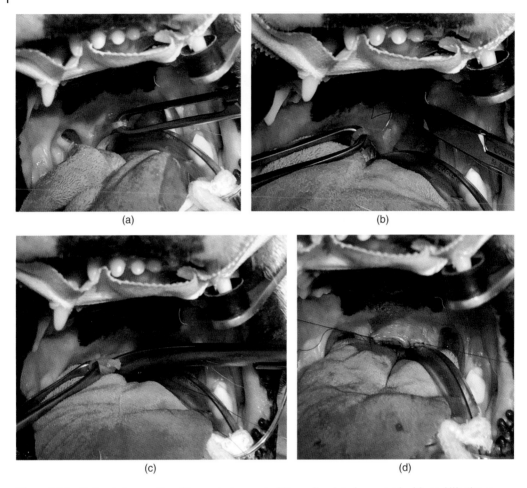

Figure 5.13 Soft palate resection. The central aspect of the soft palate is grasped with an Allis tissue forceps (a). A suture is placed at the lateral aspect of the soft palate at the desired level of resection (b). The soft palate is partially cut with Metzenbaum scissors (c) which is followed by suturing the nasal and oral epithelium until the entire soft palate is at the desired length (d).

5.10 Everted Laryngeal Saccules

Resection of the saccules is relatively simple; however it requires good visualization and delicate tissue handling to prevent post-operative swelling and edema. Increased respiratory and gastrointestinal complications have been reported in dogs after BAOS correction associated with the resection of everted laryngeal saccules [46]. A slightly undersized endotracheal tube helps with visualization as the tube can be manipulated and retracted dorsally to visualize the everted saccules without the need to remove the endotracheal tube (Figure 5.14a). The everted saccule is grasped with long Debakey, or similar, forceps and the everted saccule is transected at its base with long curved Metzenbaum scissors. The procedure is repeated on the opposite side of the larynx. Care is taken not to cut or tear the ventral aspect of the laryngeal mucosa in an effort to prevent ventral laryngeal webbing scar tissue. Hemostasis is achieved with gentle pressure with a cotton tipped applicator. The laryngeal region is gently suctioned post-procedure (Figure 5.14b).

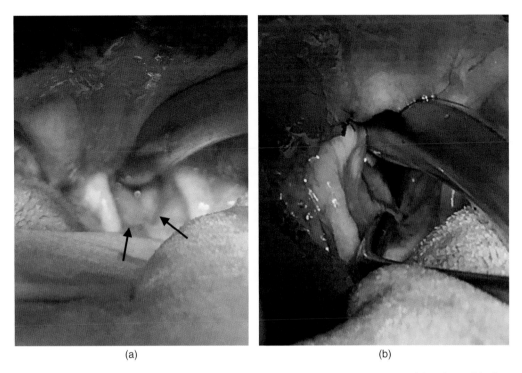

(a) (b)

Figure 5.14 (a) Bilateral everted laryngeal saccules obstructing the ventral aspect of the airway (black arrows). (b) After resection of the everted saccules. Be careful not to resect the ventral aspect of the everted laryngeal saccule mucosa to prevent scar tissue formation and ventral laryngeal webbing.

5.11 Additional Conditions

5.11.1 Epiglottic Retroversion

In cases of epiglottic retroversion, in addition to correction of an elongated soft palate, stenotic nares and everted laryngeal saccules, the epiglottis must be prevented from caudal displacement and obstruction of the rima glottidis during inspiration. Epiglottopexy can be performed as a temporary procedure, to confirm the diagnosis, or as a permanent procedure. Temporary epiglottopexy is performed by placement of several mattress sutures of 4–0 synthetic absorbable suture between the lingual surface of the epiglottis and the base of the tongue. A permanent epiglottopexy is performed by removal of the mucosa from the lingual surface of the epiglottis as well as the corresponding mucosa on the dorsal surface of the base of the tongue. Three to four mattress sutures are placed, using synthetic absorbable 3–0 or 4–0 sutures, between the central aspect of the epiglottis and the base of the tongue to fix the epiglottis in a horizontal position against the base of the tongue. The incised edge of the mucosa on the epiglottis is then sutured to the edge of the resected lingual mucosa in a simple interrupted pattern of 4–0 synthetic absorbable suture [12] (Figure 5.15). Subtotal epiglottic resection can be performed as an alternative to epiglottopexy or if there is failure of an epiglottopexy [47]. The epiglottis is grasped with long Debakey forceps and the epiglottis is cut full thickness along the widest portion of the base of the epiglottis and removed. The mucosa is sutured over the cut edge of the cartilage with fine (4–0 to 5–0) synthetic absorbable suture.

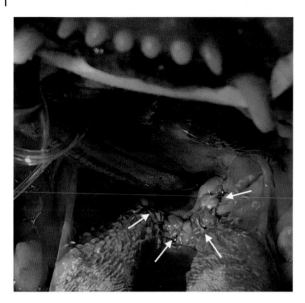

Figure 5.15 Post-operative epiglottopexy. The epiglottis is attached to the base of the tongue after removal of the ventral epiglottic and the dorsal lingual mucosa. The epiglottis is then tacked to the base of the tongue (not shown). The remaining epiglottic mucosal edge is then sutured to the edge of the resected mucosa on the base of the tongue with interrupted fine absorbable suture material (white arrows).

5.11.2   Edematous Glossoepiglottic Mucosa

Redundant edematous glossoepiglottic mucosa has been reported to entrap the epiglottis and obstruct the rima glottidis in patients with BAOS. Surgical resection of the redundant glossoepiglottic mucosa and suturing the remaining mucosa can be successful in relieving clinical signs [6].

5.11.3   Laser Assisted Turbinectomy

Aberrant turbinates have been reported as a cause of persistent diminished airflow after standard BAOS surgical procedures by restricting airflow through the nasal cavity and nasopharyngeal region [48]. These turbinates have been successfully resected with videoendoscopy aided removal with a diode laser [49, 50].

5.11.4   Temporary Tracheostomy Tube Placement

Temporary tracheostomy tubes are occasionally used with brachycephalic airway surgery if there is excessive swelling either prior to or after surgery to provide an alternate route to provide airflow. There are no objective criteria for which dogs will need a temporary tracheostomy tube after surgery, but older dogs were more likely to receive a temporary tracheostomy tube and these dogs required a longer hospital stay in one study [51]. Silicone temporary tracheostomy tubes are preferred, but an endotracheal tube can be used in an emergency situation. With the patient under anesthesia and in dorsal recumbency, a 2–3 cm skin incision is made from the caudal edge of the cricoid cartilage extending caudally. The sternohyoideus muscles are separated and retraction is maintained with Gelpi self-retaining retractors. The annular ligament between the 3rd and 4th tracheal cartilage rings is cut transversely enough to allow insertion of the tracheostomy tube. Care is taken not to extend the incision more than half the circumference of the trachea. A 2–0 suture loop is placed around the 3rd and a second loop placed around the 4th cartilage ring to allow retraction of the tracheostomy site when placing the tracheostomy tube. The endotracheal tube is then removed (if present) and the tracheostomy tube is placed. The temporary tracheostomy tube is then

Figure 5.16 A patient recovering from brachiocephalic airway surgery, alert, and tolerating the endotracheal tube.

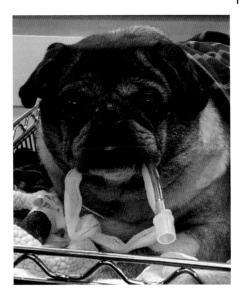

secured with either umbilical tape or sutures. Skin sutures can be placed proximal and caudal to the tracheostomy tube if the skin incision extends past the edges of the tracheostomy tube.

5.11.5 Post-operative Care

Patients recovering from upper airway surgery should be closely monitored for evidence of bleeding, laryngeal or pharyngeal edema, regurgitation, and aspiration. Patients should be allowed to remain intubated as long as possible. Brachycephalic breeds, if recovered slowly, will often tolerate the endotracheal tube until they are fully alert (Figure 5.16). If respiratory distress is noted after removal of the endotracheal tube, the patient can be reintubated or a temporary tracheostomy tube placed. Providing supplemental oxygen by mask, oxygen cage or by nasotracheal tube my help recovery and decrease the level of respiratory distress in the post-operative period [52].

Nebulization with adrenaline (0.3 mg diluted in 5 ml sterile saline) for five minutes was reported to decrease laryngeal swelling in a dog after BAOS surgery. This treatment may be appropriate in cases of post-operative upper airway swelling and further investigation is warranted [53].

The patient should be kept calm and comfortable during the recovery period. Pain management should be aimed at keeping the patient comfortable without inducing panting. Additional doses of dexamethasone (0.1–$0.2\,mg\,kg^{-1}$ IV) may be required if progressive edema is noted. The patients can be offered water 6–12 hours after the procedure and offer soft food in the form of meatballs after 12 hours [23].

Patients with temporary tracheostomy tubes should have the tubes cleaned and suctioned frequently (using sterile technique: sterile gloves, supplies, suction tubing) at least every 30–60 minutes initially, to prevent secretions from occluding the tracheostomy tube. Nebulization or instillation of small volumes (1 ml) of sterile saline into the tracheostomy tube can be used to loosen secretion followed by suctioning of the tracheostomy tube and trachea with a soft sterile suction tube [23]. The tracheostomy tubes are typically maintained for two to three days prior to removal [51].

Dogs undergoing rhinoplasty for stenotic nares should wear an Elizabethan collar to prevent self-trauma for two weeks after surgery. Patients with soft palate and laryngeal surgery should use a harness instead of a collar for at least four weeks after surgery, and possibly for life.

Brachiocephalic dogs are becoming more popular with our veterinary clients. Understanding the various aspects of treatment for BAOS and promoting early surgical intervention will improve the lives of these patients and their owners.

References

1 Lodato, D. and Hedlund, C. (2012). Brachycephalic airway syndrome: pathophysiology and diagnosis. *Compendium* 34: E1–E4.
2 Pollard, R., Johnson, L., and Marks, S. (2018). Prevalence of dynamic pharyngeal collapse is high in brachycephalic dogs undergoing videofluoroscopy. *Vet. Radiol. Ultrasound* 59: 529–534.
3 Poncet, C., Dupre, G., Freiche, V., and Bouvy, B. (2006). Long-term results of upper respiratory syndrome surgery and gastrointestinal tract medical treatment in 51 brachycephalic dogs. *J. Small Anim. Pract.* 47: 137–142.
4 Reeve, E., Sutton, D., Friend, E., and Warren-Smith, C. (2017). Documenting the prevalence of hiatal hernia and oesophageal abnormalities in brachycephalic dogs using fluoroscopy. *J. Small Anim. Pract.* 58: 703–708.
5 Arai, K., Kobayashi, M., Harada, Y. et al. (2016). Histopathologic and immunohistochemical features of soft palate muscles and nerves in dogs with an elongated soft palate. *Am. J. Vet. Res.* 77 (1): 77–83.
6 Schabbing, K. and Seaman, J. (2017). Resection and primary closure of edematous glossoepiglottic mucosa in a dog causing laryngeal obstruction. *J. Am. Anim. Hosp. Assoc.* 53: 180–184.
7 Skerrett, S., McClaran, J., Fox, P., and Palma, D. (2015). Clinical features and outcome of dogs with epiglottic retroversion with or without surgical treatment: 24 cases. *J. Vet. Intern. Med.* 29: 1611–1618.
8 De Lorenzi, D., Bertoncello, D., Mantovani, C., and Bottero, E. (2018). Nasopharyngeal sialoceles in 11 brachycephalic dogs. *Vet. Surg.* 47: 431–438.
9 Meola, S. (2013). Brachycephalic airway syndrome. *Top. Companion Anim. Med.* 28: 91–96.
10 Emmerson, T. (2014). Brachycephalic obstructive airway syndrome: a growing problem (editorial). *J. Small Anim. Pract.* 55: 543–544.
11 Fawcett, A., Barrs, V., Awad, M. et al. (2019). Consequences and management of canine brachycephaly in veterinary practice: perspectives from Australian veterinarians and veterinary specialists. *Animals* 9 (1): 1–25.
12 Flanders, J. and Thompson, M. (2009). Dyspnea caused by epiglottic retroversion in two dogs. *J. Am. Vet. Med. Assoc.* 235 (11): 1330–1335.
13 Davis, M., Cummings, S., and Payton, M. (2017). Effect of brachycephaly and body condition score on respiratory thermoregulation of healthy dogs. *J. Am. Vet. Med. Assoc.* 251 (10): 1160–1165.
14 Roedler, F., Pohl, S., and Oechtering, G. (2013). How does severe brachycephaly affect dog's lives? Results of a structured preoperative owner questionnaire. *Vet. J.* 198: 606–610.
15 Broux, O., Clercx, C., Etienne, A. et al. (2018). Effects of manipulations to detect sliding hiatal hernia in dogs with brachycephalic airway obstructive syndrome. *Vet. Surg.* 47: 243–251.
16 Kaye, B., Rutherford, L., Perridge, D., and Ter Haar, G. (2018). Relationship between brachycephalic airway syndrome and gastrointestinal signs in three breeds of dog. *J. Small Anim. Pract.* 59: 670–673.
17 Haimel, G. and Dupré, G. (2015). Brachycephalic airway syndrome: a comparative study between pugs and French bulldogs. *J. Small Anim. Pract.* 56: 714–719.

18 Riggs, J., Liu, N.-C., Sutton, D. et al. (2019). Validation of exercise testing and laryngeal auscultation for grading brachycephalic obstructive airway syndrome in pugs, French bulldogs, and English Bulldogs by using whole-body barometric plethysmography. *Vet. Surg.* 48: 1–9.

19 Evans, H. and de Lahunta, A. (2013). The respiratory system. In: *Miller's Anatomy of the Dog*, 4e, 338–361. St. Louis, MO: Elsevier.

20 Labuscagne, S., Zeiler, G., and Dzikiti, B. (2019). Effects of chemical and mechanical stimulation on laryngeal motion during alfaxalone, thiopentone or propofol anaesthesia in healthy dogs. *Vet. Anaesth.Anal.* 46: 435–442.

21 MacPhail, C. (2014). Laryngeal disease in dogs and cats. *Vet. Clin. Small Anim.* 44: 19–31.

22 Kaye, B., Boroffka, S., Haagsman, A., and Ter Haar, G. (2015). Computed tomographic, radiographic, and endoscopic tracheal dimensions in English Bulldogs with grade 1 clinical signs of brachycephalic airway syndrome. *Vet. Radiol. Ultrasound* 56 (6): 609–616.

23 MacPhail, C. (2013). Surgery of the upper respiratory system. In: *Small Animal Surgery*, 4e (ed. T. Fossum), 906–957. St. Louis, MO: Elsevier.

24 Grand, J.G. and Bureau, S. (2011). Structural characteristics of the soft palate and meatus nasopharyngeus in brachycephalic and nonbrachycephalic dogs analysed by CT. *J. Small Anim. Pract.* 52: 232–239.

25 Heidenreich, D., Gradner, G., Kneissl, S., and Dupre, G. (2016). Nasopharyngeal dimensions from computed tomography of pugs and French bulldogs with brachycephalic airway syndrome. *Vet. Surg.* 45: 83–90.

26 Liu, N., Oechtering, G., Adams, V. et al. (2017). Outcomes and prognostic factors of surgical treatments for brachycephalic obstructive airway syndrome in 3 breeds. *Vet. Surg.* 46: 271–280.

27 Rutherford, L., Beever, L., Bruce, M., and Ter Haar, G. (2017). Assessment of computed tomography derived cricoid cartilage and tracheal dimensions to evaluate degree of cricoid narrowing in brachycephalic dogs. *Vet. Radiol. Ultrasound* 58 (6): 634–646.

28 De Lorenzi, D., Bertoncello, D., and Drigo, M. (2009). Bronchial abnormalities found in a consecutive series of 40 brachycephalic dogs. *J. Am. Vet. Med. Assoc.* 235 (7): 834–840.

29 Schuenemann, R. and Oechtering, G. (2014). Inside the brachycephalic nose: intranasal mucosal contact points. *J. Am. Anim. Hosp. Assoc.* 50: 149–158.

30 Auger, M., Alexander, K., Beauchamp, G., and Dunn, M. (2016). Use of CT to evaluate and compare intranasal features in brachycephalic and normocephalic dogs. *J. Small Anim. Pract.* 57: 529–536.

31 Hoareau, G., Jourdan, G., Mellema, M., and Verwaerde, P. (2012). Evaluation of arterial blood gases and arterial blood pressures in brachycephalic dogs. *J. Vet. Intern. Med.* 26: 897–904.

32 Arulpagasam, S., Lux, C., Odunayo, A. et al. (2018). Evaluation of pulse oximetry in healthy brachycephalic dogs. *J. Am. Anim. Hosp. Assoc.* 54: 34–350.

33 Hostnik, E., Scansen, B., Zielinski, R., and Ghadiali, S. (2017). Quantification of nasal airflow resistance in English Bulldogs using computed tomography and computational fluid dynamics. *Vet. Radiol. Ultrasound* 58: 542–551.

34 Hinchliffe, T., Liu, N., and Ladlow, J. (2019). Sleep-disordered breathing in the Cavalier King Charles spaniel: a case series. *Vet. Surg.* 48: 497–504.

35 Liu, N., Adams, V., Kalmar, L. et al. (2016). Whole-body barometric plethysmography characterizes upper airway obstruction in 3 brachycephalic breeds of dogs. *J. Vet. Intern. Med.* 30: 853–865.

36 Riecks, T., Birchard, S., and Stephens, J. (2007). Surgical correction of brachycephalic syndrome in dogs: 62 cases (1991-2004). *J. Am. Vet. Med. Assoc.* 230 (9): 1324–1328.

37 Bersenas, A., Mathews, K., Allen, D., and Conlon, P. (2005). Effects of ranitidine, famotidine, pantoprazole, and omeprazole on intragastric pH in dogs. *Am. J. Vet. Res.* 66: 425–431.

38 Veasey, S., Fenik, P., Panckeri, K. et al. (1999). The effects of trazodone with L-tryptophan on sleep disordered breathing in the English Bulldog. *Am. J. Respir. Crit. Care Med.* 160: 1659–1667.

39 Huck, J., Stanley, B., and Hauptman, J. (2008). Technique and outcome of nares amputation (Trader's technique) in immature shih tzus. *J. Am. Anim. Hosp. Assoc.* 44 (2): 82–85.

40 Monnet, E. (2004). Brachycephalic airway syndrome. In: *Textbook of Small Animal Surgery*, 3e (ed. D. Slatter), 808–813. Philadelphia, PA: Saunders.

41 Trostel, C.T. and Frankel, D. (2010). Punch resection alaplasty technique in dogs and cats with stenotic nares: 14 cases. *J. Am. Anim. Hosp. Assoc.* 46 (1): 5–11.

42 Clark, G. and Sinibaldi, K. (1994). Use of carbon dioxide laser for treatment of elongated soft palate in dogs. *J. Am. Vet. Med. Assoc.* 204 (11): 1779–1781.

43 Kirsch, M., Spector, D., Kalafut, S. et al. (2019). Comparison of carbon dioxide laser vs bipolar vessel sealing device for staphylectomy for the treatment of brachycephalic airway obstructive airway syndrome. *Can. Vet. J.* 60: 160–166.

44 Brdecka, D., Rawlings, C., Howerth, E. et al. (2007). A histopathological comparison of two techniques for soft palate resection in normal dogs. *Am. Anim. Hosp. Assoc.* 43: 39–44.

45 Findji, L. and Dupré, G. (2008). Folded flap palatoplasty for treatment of elongated soft palates in 55 dogs. *Wien. Tierärztl. Mschr.* 95: 56–63.

46 Hughes, J., Kaye, B., Beswick, A., and Ter Haar, G. (2018). Complications following laryngeal sacculectomy in brachycephalic dogs. *J. Small Anim. Pract.* 59: 16–21.

47 Mullins, R., McAlinden, A., and Goodfellow, M. (2014). Subtotal epiglottectomy for the management of epiglottic retroversion in a dog. *J. Small Anim. Pract.* 55: 383–385.

48 Vilaplana, G., Haar, G., and Boroffka, S. (2015). Gender, weight, and age effects on prevalence of caudal aberrant nasal turbinates in clinically healthy English Bulldogs: a computed tomographic study and classification. *Vet. Radiol. Ultrasound* 56: 486–493.

49 Oechtering, G., Pohl, S., Schlueter, C. et al. (2016). A novel approach to brachycephalic syndrome. 2. Laser-assisted turbinectomy (LATE). *Vet. Surg.* 45: 173–181.

50 Schuenemann, R., Pohl, S., and Oechtering, G. (2017). A novel approach to brachycephalic syndrome. 3. Isolated laser-assisted turbinectomy of caudal aberrant turbinates (CAT LATE). *Vet. Surg.* 46: 32–38.

51 Worth, D., Grimes, J., Jiménez, D. et al. (2018). Risk factors for temporary tracheostomy tube placement following surgery to alleviate signs of brachycephalic obstructive airway syndrome in dogs. *J. Am. Vet. Med. Assoc.* 253: 1158–1163.

52 Senn, D., Sigrist, N., Forterre, F. et al. (2011). Retrospective evaluation of post-operative nasotracheal tubes for oxygen supplementation in dogs following surgery for brachycephalic syndrome: 36 cases (2003–2007). *J. Vet. Emerg. Crit. Care* 21 (3): 261–267.

53 Ellis, J. and Leece, E. (2017). Nebulized adrenaline in the postoperative management of brachycephalic obstructive airway syndrome in a pug. *J. Am. Anim. Hosp. Assoc.* 53: 107–110.

6

The Unique Welfare Challenges of Brachycephalism

Kymberley C. McLeod

Conundrum Consulting, Toronto, Ontario, Canada

The ownership of breeds with brachycephalic head structure has grown faster than any other variety of dog over the last decade, making up eight of the top 32 American Kennel Club (AKC) breeds [1]. According to the AKC, the French Bulldog has climbed from 52nd in 2003 to 4th largest breed by registrations in 2019, with the English Bulldog right behind at number 5. Brachycephalic breeds also comprise three of the top six most popular breeds in the United Kingdom [2]. Meaning "shortened head," brachycephalic breeds have a distinctly short nose and flattened facial shape. While small breeds, such as Pugs and Shih Tzus, are most commonly thought of when discussing brachycephalic breeds, we must remember that the conformation is also exhibited in larger breeds such as Chow Chows and Bulldogs.

With their drastic rise in popularity, awareness of the unique set of welfare challenges to patients born within this phenotype has been growing. There are currently several campaigns [3–7] to stop or change how we are breeding these dogs directly due to these welfare concerns. In this chapter, we will detail how brachycephalic dogs may experience increased amounts of oral and skeletal pain, oral infection, emotional/physical distress and an altered ability to express natural behaviors, simply due to their purposefully chosen confirmation. Further, while the effects of these welfare-compromising concerns may seem to present acutely (if noticed at all), the affected state is generally chronic and present from birth. This may continue despite recommended interventional surgery, even when clinical signs are reduced [8] (see Chapter 5). Ethically, the veterinary profession needs to understand that while these abnormalities may be extraordinarily common within these breeds, they are not normal nor desirable [9, 10]. Assessing every animal of brachycephalic conformation for welfare-related challenges should become routine in the veterinary exam, and where necessary, it is our ethical duty to advocate for appropriate therapeutic interventions. Additionally, providing education and assistance to breeders and owners of brachycephalic animals about the welfare challenges of brachycephalic breeds may help guide improved choices within the breeding and owner communities [11].

6.1 Oral Infection

There is widespread evidence linking extreme brachycephalic phenotypes with chronic disease [12]. Insurance claims for both acute and chronic disease in brachycephalics far outnumber claims made by other popular breeds [13]. As has been noted in the previous chapters, when left untreated,

Breed Predispositions to Dental and Oral Disease in Dogs, First Edition. Edited by Brook A. Niemiec.
© 2021 John Wiley & Sons, Inc. Published 2021 by John Wiley & Sons, Inc.

dental infections create both serious local and systemic effects, and their deleterious physiological drain is a significant welfare concern for the patient.

Chronic periodontal disease risk is significantly increased in small and brachycephalic breeds in part due to tooth crowding and rotation [14–19]. Their proportionally larger teeth and small jaws (compared with larger breed dogs), increased propensity to retain deciduous teeth, and decreased bone quality of the rostral mandible quicken onset of disease, as well as worsen total lifetime severity [20, 21].

While the recommendation in Chapter 2 of preventive extraction in the face of crowding to prevent more serious negative outcomes may seem radical to some practitioners, preventive surgery for welfare benefits occurs relatively regularly in the veterinary profession. Most notable is the routine use of preventive sterilization to lessen the chance of sex hormone related cancers. When excessive crowding of the cheek teeth occurs in brachycephalics, delaying or avoiding treatment can result in the extraction of both teeth due to periodontal disease [19]. This leaves the patient to suffer the effects of pain and infection, as well as loss of chewing function of the affected teeth forever. In contrast, addressing crowding or rotational based concerns preventively can decrease the likelihood and/or severity of periodontal disease, allowing for retention of the more functionally beneficial tooth [19]. This approach of balancing of welfare needs to maximize overall welfare during a patient's lifetime fits into the utilitarian model [22] of animal welfare and is very applicable to veterinary care decision making.

Likewise, there is a distinct increase in the incidence of non-eruption and tooth impaction in brachycephalic breeds. Impacted teeth are often painful in humans (and thus presumably in dogs), and can lead to malignant transformation, or dangerous dentigerous cysts, which may get infected and/or cause pathologic jaw fractures [23–28]. While the rate of occurrence is high, the understanding that deleterious effects can occur when no tooth appears present in its anatomically appropriate location is reported anecdotally to be quite lacking. Radiographic examination of any non-erupted teeth should be done as soon as a missing tooth is noted, to ensure it is not painfully impacted or fractured below the gumline [25, 26].

6.2 Oral Pain

When humans selectively breed for extremes in conformation, unexpected deleterious effects to the welfare of those animals may become evident over time. Purposeful malocclusions in small and brachycephalic breeds can compromise daily welfare for animals with this extreme conformation. No matter whether the animal is "eating normally" or not, trauma to teeth or oral tissues that occurs during routine closing of the mouth requires appropriate therapy. The pain experienced with this type of trauma is significant and constant, and as such ethically requires the veterinarian to take action to remove the source of this pain. The consequences of leaving teeth that traumatically contact other teeth or the soft tissues of the oral cavity are not benign. Over time, tissue ulceration, enamel attrition and dentin exposure, fracture, traumatic pulpitis, endodontic disease, and abscessation are all expected consequences, and each carry significant, chronic, and wholly avoidable pain [29–32]. As has been previously stated, pain cannot be seen on radiographs or other advanced imaging options, but when reasonably suspected, must be addressed. A lack of change in appetite is not adequate evidence that oral pain is not occurring.

6.3   Emotional/Physical Distress

As has been previously described in Chapter 5, brachycephalic conformation has created decreased maxillary length without proportional decrease in soft tissue structures of the nasal cavity and pharynx. This inadvertent anatomical excess of soft tissue contributes to a syndrome commonly referred to as brachycephalic obstructive airway syndrome (BOAS) [33]. Many brachycephalic breeds are affected, with English and French Bulldogs, Pugs, and Boston Terriers being the most common. Some breeds estimate 70–75% prevalence of BOAS within all individuals surveyed [9].

The varying degrees of upper airway dysfunction and obstruction create the need for excessive breathing effort simply to move air in and out of the body. Over time, this increased breathing effort can lead to laryngeal collapse, hypotrophy of the pharyngeal muscles, and/or eversion of the tonsils, further narrowing the upper airways [33]. In other words, the simple, survival-driven act of drawing each moment's breath is the very activity that contributes to greater effort being required to take the next.

This syndrome is most commonly diagnosed in young adults, however the welfare impacts of this syndrome are life long and significant, and may reduce overall quality of life (QOL) for those affected. The ability to breathe is essential for survival, and dogs with BOAS suffer great distress from air starvation, and possibly fear and anxiety when facing respiratory distress. Breathlessness or air starvation compromises welfare in multifactorial ways [34]. In human medicine, air hunger, respiratory effort, and chest tightness are separately recognized causes of breathlessness, with air hunger being reported to be the most stressful and unpleasant. For brachycephalic dogs, the cerebral cortical processing reflects increased respiratory effort even at rest, and true air hunger during even mild exertion [35]. Heat and exercise intolerance directly linked to this inability to breathe have been reported.

6.4   Other Health and Behavior-Related Concerns

Outside of oral and nasal concerns, brachycephalic dogs seem to show higher incidences of other types of disease as well. A higher prevalence of ocular disease was noted, with corneal ulceration being three to four times more common than in breeds with other facial structures. Additionally, increases in conjunctivitis and corneal trauma were all noted.

The foreshortening of the muzzle has created excessive skin folding in many of these breeds, with increased rates of dermal disease being reported. Other concerns with increased prevalence include digestive disorders, urinary tract infections, pneumonia, and respiratory distress [13].

Research shows that when animals face significant levels of negative welfare, this discomfort leads to less central motivation to engage in more rewarding, positive behaviors. Without the ability to breathe comfortably and easily at rest and during physical activity, their ability to express behaviors as simple as exercise and play behavior can be severely affected. For some, severe respiratory crisis can be brought on by simply walking outside in humid weather [9].

The lack of exercise makes obesity prevention particularly challenging. Obesity has several deleterious effects on quality and quantity of life, reducing lifespan in some studies by up to 2.5 years [36]. Obesity also leads to extra physical fat deposition around the upper airways, resulting in increased respiratory distress. Other potential side effects of obesity, such as increased propensity to degenerative joint disease and the pain associated with this chronic inflammatory condition, must not be discounted [37].

6.5 Normalization

Heritable diseases like brachycephalism present a frustrating challenge when talking with veterinary clients for both general practitioners and specialists alike. This is because common phenotypic welfare challenges may be seen as "normal" for the breed, and therefore not valid or concerning to the owner. There is a large difference, however, between common and normal. Packer et al. [38] reported that in a large multicentric study of brachycephalic breed owners, 58% of them did not feel that the signs of breathing difficulty identified in their own pet by a specialist were an issue, but instead "normal" for their pet.

The concept of "normalization" explains the change of perception that occurs over time until signs of disease no longer appear abnormal, due to either large proportions of animals within breeds showing these clinical signs, and/or the animal themselves has always seemed to exhibit that behavior. Sadly, normalization leads to a percentage of pet parents and veterinarians that will not self-identify these conditions as pathological, nor consider them reasons to seek or recommend therapeutic care. This may also leave these animals in the breeding pool to continue passing along their genetic material to future generations. Therefore, continuing to educate brachycephalic owners that "common" isn't necessarily "normal" L is essential.

6.6 Effects on Quality of Life (QOL)

The ability to adequately manage pain and infection on a day-to-day basis are central tenets of most of the currently utilized QOL assessment rubrics available to small animal practitioners [39, 40]. While QOL assessment may occur to an owner making end of life decisions, it is far less commonly discussed when brachycephalic puppies or young adults appear in the veterinary clinical setting. When we look logically at QOL assessment tools, these can be usefully applied at any age to help guide a client as to when additional veterinary support should be sought out for their pet.

In the dental context, while a single mode of therapy may be started at an early age (i.e. home care), if the animal's need for therapy outstrips the ability of the prescribed prevention to prevent disease progression (i.e. gingivitis progresses to periodontal disease), QOL for that patient begins to suffer. Clients need to understand when to return for additional help. Predictive education should be included with prescriptive solutions to assist clients in understanding how to evaluate clinical success of recommendations. When clients feel unsure as to their ability to assess or monitor efficacy, the veterinary healthcare team can be mobilized to provide this in the form of regular rechecks.

The last two decades have brought much media and public attention to the consequences of human intervention into selective dog breeding for performance, behavior or appearance. Driving this change are passionate voices in both the veterinary and academic worlds. By educating our prospective and current pet parents and breeders on the welfare consequences of these diseases, we continue to amplify the message. Every individual animal challenged by its own conformation deserves to have its needs assessed and addressed, to allow for the best possible daily welfare. Dogs with a brachycephalic conformation have a disproportionately higher likelihood to suffer from welfare affecting conditions specifically due to the purposeful breeding for this conformation. If a large majority of the breed shows compromise in least one of the Five Animal Welfare Needs (see Chapter 3), then by both utilitarian and deontological ethical frameworks, encouraging breeding for this conformation is ethically unacceptable [12].

References

1 American Kennel Club (2018). Most popular breeds. www.akc.org/most-popular-breeds (accessed 20 June 2020).

2 Humane Society Veterinary Medical Association (2018). Fact sheet. Health and welfare issues associated with brachycephalic dogs. https://hsvma.memberclicks.net/assets/pdfs/Fact%20 %20Sheet%20-%20Brachycephalics.pdf (accessed 20 June 2020).

3 Wedderburn, P. (2016). Urgent call by vet profession to stop suffering of brachycephalic dogs and cats. https://vethelpdirect.com/vetblog/2016/05/09/vets-to-end-suffering-of-brachycephalic-dogs/# (accessed 20 June 2020).

4 Evans, M. (2018). Continuing the campaign on brachycephalic dogs. *Vet. Rec.* 182: 114.

5 British Veterinary Association. (2020). All animals should be bred for health over looks. www .bva.co.uk/take-action/breed-to-breathe-campaign (accessed 20 June 2020).

6 Vets on the Balkans (2018). Brachycephalic and flat-faced breeds. http://balkanvets.com/index. php/tag/brachycephalic-flat-faced-breeds (accessed 20 June 2020).

7 Hale, F. (2013). Stop brachycephalism, now! *Can. Vet. J.* 54 (2): 185–186.

8 Pohl, S., Roedler, F.S., and Oechtering, G.U. (2016). How does multilevel upper airway surgery influence the lives of dogs with severe brachycephaly? Results of a structured pre- and postoperative owner questionnaire. *Vet. J.* 210: 39–45.

9 Packer, R.M.A., Hendricks, A., Tivers, M.S., and Burn, C.C. (2015). Impact of facial conformation on canine health: brachycephalic obstructive airway syndrome. *PLoS One* 10 (10): e0137496. https://doi.org/10.1371/journal.pone.0137496.

10 Roedler, F.S., Pohl, S., and Oechtering, G.U. (2013). How does severe brachycephaly affect dog's lives? Results of a structured preoperative owner questionnaire. *Vet. J.* 198 (3): 606–610.

11 Steinert, K., Kuhne, F., Kramer, M., and Hackbarth, H. (2019). People's perception of brachycephalic breeds and breed-related welfare problems in Germany. *J. Vet. Behav.* 33: 96–102.

12 Fawcett, A., Barrs, V., Awad, M. et al. (2018). Consequences and management of canine brachycephaly in veterinary practice: perspectives from Australian veterinarians and veterinary specialists. *Animals* 9 (1): 3. https://doi.org/10.3390/ani9010003.

13 Feng, T., McConnell, C., O'Hara, K. et al. (2017). Nationwide's brachycephalic breed disease prevalence study. http://nationwidedvm.com/wp-content/uploads/2017/03 NWBrachycelphalic-Study0317.pdf (accessed 20 June 2020).

14 Hale, F.A. (2005). Juvenile veterinary dentistry. *Vet. Clin. Small Anim.* 35: 789–817.

15 Hennet, P.R. and Harvey, C.E. (1992). Craniofacial development and growth in the dog. *J. Vet. Dent.* 9 (2): 11–18.

16 Wetering, A.V. (2011). Dental and oral cavity. In: *Small Animal Pediatrics* (eds. M.E. Peterson and M.A. Kutzler), 340–348. St. Louis, MO: Elsevier.

17 Debowes, L.J. (2010). Problems with the gingiva. In: *Small Animal Dental, Oral and Maxillofacial Disease, a Color Handbook* (ed. B.A. Niemiec), 159–181. London: Manson.

18 Buckley, L.A. (1972). The relationship between malocclusion and periodontal disease. *J. Periodontol.* 43 (7): 415–417.

19 Startup, S. (2013). Rotated, crowded, and supernummery teeth. In: *Veterinary Orthodontics* (ed. B.A. Niemiec), 66–72. Tustin: Practical Veterinary Publishing.

20 Niemiec, B.A. (2013). Pathogenesis and etiology of periodontal disease. In: *Veterinary Periodontology* (ed. B.A. Niemiec), 18–34. Ames: Wiley Blackwell.

21 Alsulaiman, A.A., Kaye, E., Jones, J. et al. (2018). Incisor malalignment and the risk of periodontal disease progression. *Am. J. Orthod. Dentofacial. Orthop.* 153 (4): 512–522.

22 Palmer, C. and Sandoe, P. (2018). Animal ethics. In: *Animal Welfare*, 3e (eds. M. Appleby, A. Olsson and F. Galindo), 3–16. CABI.

23 Fulton, A. and Fiani, N. (2011). Diagnostic imaging in veterinary dental practice. Dentigerous cyst with secondary infection. *J. Am. Vet. Med. Assoc.* 238 (4): 435–437.

24 Niemiec, B.A. (2010). Pathology in the pediatric patient. In: *Small Animal Dental Oral and Maxillofacial Disease* (ed. B.A. Niemeic), 89–126. London, UK: Manson.

25 Niemiec, B.A. (2011). The importance of dental radiology. *Eur. J. Comp. Anim. Pract.* 20 (3): 219–229.

26 Niemiec, B.A. (2017). The importance of and indications for dental radiology. In: *Practical Veterinary Dental Radiology* (eds. B.A. Niemiec, J. Gawor and V. Jekel), 5–30. CRC Press.

27 Grisar, K., Schol, M., Hauben, E. et al. (2016). Primary intraosseous squamous cell carcinoma of the mandible arising from an infected odontogenic cyst: a case report and review of the literature. *Oncol. Lett.* 12 (6): 5327–5331.

28 Bellows, J. (2004). Oral surgical equipment, materials, and techniques. In: *Small Animal Dental Equipment, Materials, and Techniques, a Primer*, 297–361. Blackwell.

29 Dupont, G. (2010). Pathologies of the dental hard tissues. In: *Small Animal Dental, Oral and Maxillofacial Disease-a Color Handbook* (ed. B.A. Niemiec), 128–159. London: Manson.

30 Niemiec, B.A. (2005). Fundamentals of endodontics. *Vet. Clin. North Am. Small Anim. Pract.* 35 (4): 837–868.

31 Niemiec, B.A. (2008). Oral pathology. *Top. Companion Anim. Med.* 23 (2): 59–71.

32 Startup, S. (2011). Tooth defense and response. In: *Veterinary Endodontics* (ed. B.A. Niemiec), 16–36. Tustin: Practical Veterinary Publishing.

33 Clarke, D.L. (2015). Upper airway disease. In: *Small Animal Critical Care Medicine* (eds. D.C. Silverstein and K. Hopper), 92–104. St Louis: Saunders.

34 Broom, D.M. and Johnson, K.G. (2019). Assessing welfare: short-term responses. In: *Stress and Animal Welfare*, 99–130. Springer.

35 Beausoleil, N.J. and Mellor, D.J. (2015). Introducing breathlessness as a significant animal welfare issue. *N. Z. Vet. J.* 63 (1): 44–51.

36 Salt, C., Morris, P.J., Wilson, D. et al. (2019). Association between life span and body condition in neutered client-owned dogs. *J. Vet. Intern. Med.* 33 (1): 89–99.

37 German, A. (2006). The growing problem of obesity in dogs and cats. *J. Nutr.* 136 (7): 1940–1946.

38 Packer, R.M.A., Hendricks, A., and Burn, C.C. (2012). Do dog owners perceive the clinical signs related to conformational inherited disorders as 'normal' for the breed? A potential constraint to improving canine welfare. *Anim. Welfare* 21: 81–93.

39 Belshaw, Z., Asher, L., Harvey, N., and Dean, R. (2015). Quality of life assessment in domestic dogs: an evidence-based rapid review. *Vet. J.* 206 (2): 203–212.

40 Spitznagel, M., Jacobson, D., Cox, M., and Carlson, M. (2018). Predicting caregiver burden in general veterinary clients: contribution of companion animal clinical signs and problem behaviors. *Vet. J.* 236: 23–30.

7

Other Heritable Conditions

Brook A. Niemiec

Veterinary Dental Specialties and Oral Surgery, San Diego, CA, USA

7.1 Mandibular Canine Linguoversion (Base Narrow Canines)

Linguoversed (base narrow) mandibular canines is a fairly common issue in dogs [1–4]. This is a class 1 malocclusion, where the front to back spacing is normal, but a tooth or teeth are out of position [5]. Class 1 malocclusions may be non-genetic, however doliocephalic breeds (Collies, Airedales) as well as narrow jawed dogs are overrepresented [6, 7]. The doliocephalic head shape is defined as patients with a long and narrow head [8].

It was previously held that this condition was caused by a persistent deciduous tooth [9]. However, it is now known that the deciduous tooth becomes persistent because the permanent tooth followed an incorrect eruption path (see retained deciduous teeth) [6]. The deciduous tooth, however, will hold the permanent in the incorrect position and thus should be extracted expediently [7].

In general, there are no clinical signs associated with the malocclusion as dogs very rarely show outward evidence of the condition. However, the malocclusion generally creates significant trauma, generally to the palate, but on occasion to the gingiva and teeth (Figure 7.1). Clinical signs which *may* be associated with the condition include [7]:

- Ptyalism
- Partial anorexia or quidding
- Head shyness and less interest in playing
- In advanced cases sneezing may be seen secondary to an oronasal fistula (see below).

While we know that this condition is quite painful for the patient, there are other more significant potential sequelae to this condition which may include [5, 6, 10]:

- There is almost always palatine trauma, but gingival/tooth is also possible.
- The constant damage to the palate can eventually result in an oronasal fistula (Figure 7.2).
- The concussive trauma to the teeth can result in tooth death and endodontic infection. (Figure 7.3).

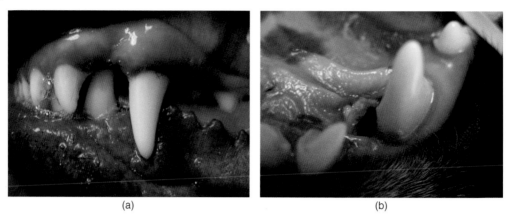

(a)   (b)

Figure 7.1 (a) Linguoversed left mandibular canine (304) in a Collie from the buccal aspect. (b) Significant palatine trauma from the maloccluded canine in (a) above.

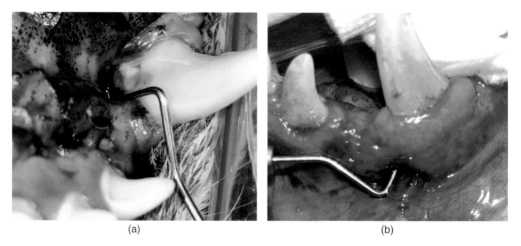

(a)   (b)

Figure 7.2 Oronasal fistula which occurred secondary to a linguoversed mandibular canine. Note that the patient also has a class II malocclusion (MAL). (a) Ventrodorsal view of the palate showing the probe in the nasal cavity, confirming the oronasal fistula. (b) Lateral view of the patient showing the buccal draining tract from the infected area.

7.1.1 Therapy for Linguoversion of the Deciduous Canines

This malocclusion is generally present in the deciduous teeth, and can typically be diagnosed as early as four weeks of age [7, 11].

Early diagnosis and treatment of this condition is important for two reasons. First, deciduous canines are significantly sharper than the permanent and create painful holes in the palate [7] (Figure 7.4). Second, the cusp tips of the deciduous canines are held in the hole they created. This will not allow the jaw to grow to its full genetic potential, typically leading to a malocclusion in the permanent dentition [5, 6] (Figure 7.5).

While coronal amputation and vital pulp therapy has been mentioned as a treatment option [12], this author prefers extraction of the offending deciduous canine(s) [6]. Extractions of deciduous canines must be performed with patience and care to avoid damaging the permanent counterpart (see persistent deciduous teeth).

Figure 7.3 Intrinsically stained (discolored) left mandibular canine (304) in a dog with a linguocclusion. This tooth is non-vital and must be treated with root canal therapy or extraction.

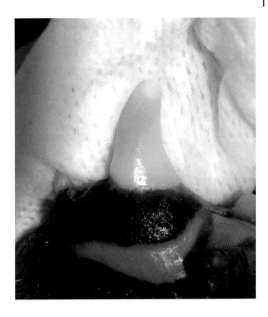

Figure 7.4 Intraoral dental picture of a patient with bilateral linguocclused deciduous mandibular canines (704 and 804) revealing significant damage. In addition, there is purulent discharge from the defects, indicating local infection.

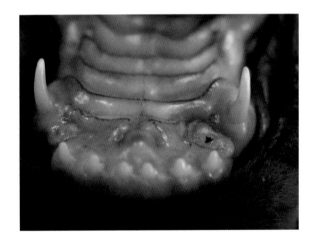

7.1.2 Treatment of Permanent Mandibular Canine Linguoversion

A plethora of therapeutic options exist for this condition, including:

- Rubber ball therapy
- Gingival wedge
- Composite extensions
- Extraction
- Crown reduction and vital pulp therapy
- Orthodontic tooth movement (incline planes).

While surgical tooth repositioning and active force orthodontics have been described, it is not recommended by this author [13–15].

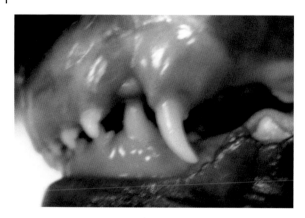

Figure 7.5 Left lateral image of the patient in (Figure 7.4). The canine is held lingually by the palatine defect. Early extraction (interceptive orthodontics) (6–8 weeks of age) may allow for the buccal movement of the teeth.

7.1.3 Repositioning (Orthodontic) Options

All of these options are based on the assumption that linguoversion is the only malocclusion. If additional orthodontic issues create impedance to tipping the tooth buccally (most commonly a class II malocclusion) these techniques become much more challenging to impossible to perform. In these cases, coronal amputation and vital pulp therapy or extraction is preferred. One major advantage to orthodontically treating these teeth is that once the canines are buccal to the maxilla, the maxilla acts as a natural retainer. Therefore, the appliances can be removed earlier, without the risk of rebound.

7.1.3.1 Mild Cases with Therapy Initiated Prior to Complete Tooth Eruption
Rubber Ball Therapy
This technique employs a rubber ball which fits the mouth well and is big enough to exert lateral pressure on the mandibular canines [7, 16]. The pet must chew on the ball for a minimum of 15 minutes three times per day until the occlusion is correct. The main advantage of this form of therapy is that no anesthesia is required. However, it is only effective on young dogs who are orally active and have a mild malocclusion. The author has had poor success with this technique.

Gingival Wedge
Creating a gingival wedge (Figure 7.6) is generally performed with a coarse diamond bur on an air-driven high-speed handpiece [7, 17, 18]. Using the gingival or palatine trauma as a starting point (a), the gingival tissue is removed to create a ramp for the canine to slide out buccally (b). This procedure only requires a single anesthesia to complete. However, it is only effective in very mild cases as only a small amount of tissue can be removed. While making a flap and removing maxillary bone to create a larger wedge has been reported [10], this author would opt for an incline plane in these cases.

Composite Crown Extensions
This is a form of an incline plane, but uses the maxillary diastema and extended crowns as the orthodontic appliance [7, 19]. As with the other techniques above, this procedure will only be effective in mild cases and during eruption. The extended teeth are quite easy to fracture, due to the leverage arm created. This technique requires two anesthesias (application and removal).

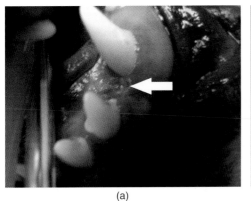
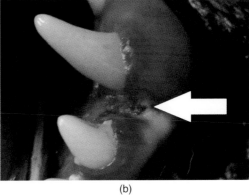

(a)   (b)

Figure 7.6   Gingival wedge to correct a minor linguoclusion. (a) Pre-operative picture revealing the minor trauma (white arrow). (b) Post-operative picture of the gingival wedge (white arrow).

The cusp tips of the mandibular canines are extended in a buccal direction. An acid etched bonding agent is applied to the cusp tips creating a crown extension (Figure 7.7). The teeth are tilted labially when the mouth is closed and the extensions contact the gingiva.

Figure 7.7   Composite extension applied to a mandibular left canine (304) to direct the tooth labially.

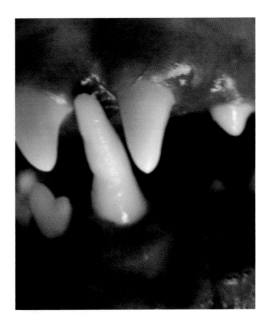

7.1.4   For Large Discrepancies or When Treatment is Starting Following Complete Canine Eruption

7.1.4.1   Incline Planes

These appliances exert a tipping force on the lingual surface of the crown of the mandibular canine in an attempt to tilt the tooth labially on its long axis in a labial direction [1, 2, 4, 5, 15, 20]. These provide intermittent force, which may be safer than constant force options as the patient self-regulates the force applied. However, constant force may work faster, but increases the risk of damage. Remember, in cases of unilateral linguoclusion, the appliance must be created to contact both mandibular canines to prevent a reflex rotation of the jaw [6, 7]. Typically the appliance is maintained for four weeks, but treatment could range from two to eight weeks [2, 17].

7.1.4.2 Acrylic Incline Plane

This is the preferred type of incline plane by most veterinary dentists [1, 2, 7, 17]. The main reason is that it is created in the mouth, thus allowing for therapy to be completed in just two anesthetic events (application and removal). This decreases the cost, as does the fact that there are no laboratory fees for fabrication. However, experience is necessary to properly bond the appliance as well as to create the correct incline and position of the ramp. In addition, the acrylic can be broken by the patient (especially orally active large breed dogs).

Several options exist for the creation of these appliances. The first two start with acid etching and then applying the acrylic directly on the teeth to be included in the splint. Following hardening, the splint is shaped and smoothed with burs.

- Two separate units between the ipsilateral maxillary canine and third incisors (Figure 7.8):
  a. Smaller and weaker
  b. Allows maxillary growth
  c. Best for small breed and/or young patients
- One large device can be created which connects the canines and covers the palate (Figure 7.9):
  a. Stronger but has more acrylic in mouth
     - Increases risk of palatitis [21].
  b. Growth of the maxilla is restricted, unless a telescoping spacer is placed
     - Weakens the appliance.
  c. Best for large breeds and patients over eight months of age.
- A variation of the single piece appliance is to place the acrylic on the teeth and allow it to harden. Then the appliance is removed and shaped outside of the mouth. Once it is properly designed, it is bonded to the maxillary canines with a dental bonding agent [22] (Figure 7.10). The major advantages to this technique are:
- Less debris in the oral cavity
- Strong bond with the tooth
- Decreased risk of damaging the teeth during shaping
- The technician could be performing other oral tasks while the veterinarian shapes the appliance

7.1.4.3 Cast Metal Incline Plane (Mann)

See (Figure 7.11). This appliance [3, 6, 23] is created by a crown or orthodontic laboratory from full mouth impressions [5]. Therefore, the veterinarian must create precise alginate impressions and bite registration. Next, they must pour and safely deliver the stone modes to the laboratory. When the appliance is returned, it is cemented to the maxillary canines.

This choice has several advantages over other methods, including (Figure 7.11):

1. The lab creates the device, ensuring proper fit and angle of ramp.
2. It is smaller, which decreases soft tissue inflammation.
3. It is much stronger than acrylic.
4. Typically, a telescoping bar is added, allowing for maxillary growth.

Figure 7.8 Two-piece direct acrylic splint attached to the canines distally and second and third incisors mesially to the diastema.

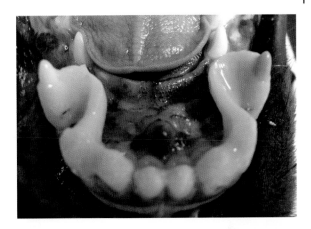

Figure 7.9 One-piece direct incline plane fabricated with dental acrylic which bridges the canines.

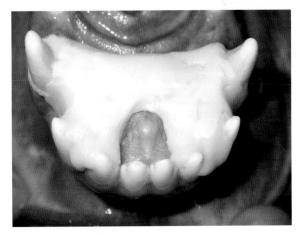

The only advantages to the acrylic versions are that they are cheaper and only require two anesthetic events. The cast metal requires three (impressions, installation, removal).

On occasion, orthodontic movement may not be the best choice. This may be because the patent is older or too orally active. The movement may be complicated by a hindrance to labial tipping due to class II malocclusion or a mesioclused maxillary canine. Finally, the client may wish for therapy to be completed in one visit (due to distance or schedule). In these cases, removing the source of trauma in one visit may be prudent. This can be via removing the entire tooth, or the cusp tip which is creating the trauma.

7.1.4.4 Coronal Amputation and Vital Pulp Therapy

This technique (see Figure 7.12) is preferred to extraction because it removes the source of trauma while being far less invasive than extraction [6, 24–26]. It also maintains most of the tooth structure to allow proper function as well as hold the tongue in the mouth. However, there is a small risk of future tooth death and infection, and thus regular radiographic monitoring (under general anesthesia) is required.

7.1.4.5 Extraction

The final and most extreme option for this condition is extraction [2, 16, 26, 27]. However, this is a very difficult procedure due to the length and curve of the root. Furthermore, mandibular

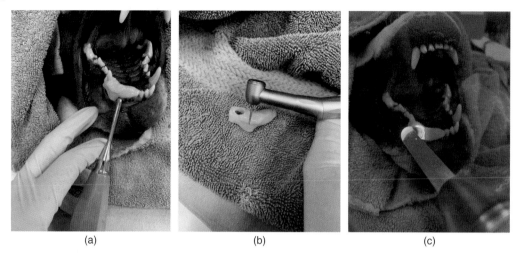

(a)   (b)   (c)

Figure 7.10 The Furman technique of incline plane application. (Note that the plane needs to be bilateral to avoid shifting.) (a) The acrylic is applied to the teeth to be included in the splint without etching the teeth and roughly shaped. Then it is carefully removed with an elevator. (b) The incline plane is shaped and smoothed with an acrylic or diamond bur. (c) The plane is cemented into place with a dental bonding agent and light cured. Source: Courtesy of Dr. Robert Furman DAVDC.

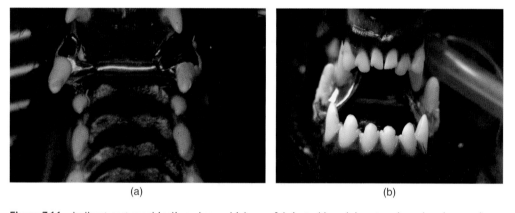

(a)   (b)

Figure 7.11 Indirect cast meal incline plane which was fabricated by a laboratory based on impressions and stone models which has been cemented on to the maxillary canines. (a) Ventral view and (b) rostral view.

canines make up approximately 60–70% of the mandible [28], This makes idiopathic mandibular fractures during extractions much more likely [29] (Figure 7.13). In addition, wound dehiscence is a common complication. Dogs utilize their canines for picking up objects (like fingers) and they maintain tongue position. Therefore, this should be considered the last option of therapy.

7.1.4.6 Mesioclused Maxillary Canines (Lance Effect)

This malocclusion is most common in the Shetland Sheepdog, but is also seen in Dachshunds, Collies, and Italian Greyhounds [5, 30]. This is a class I malocclusion, where the maxilla and mandible are of the proper length, but the maxillary canines are mesiocclused (pointing forward) [5, 31].The mesioversion was previously thought to be caused by delayed exfoliation of the deciduous canine teeth since the permanent tooth erupts mesial to the deciduous [30]. While this may rarely be the

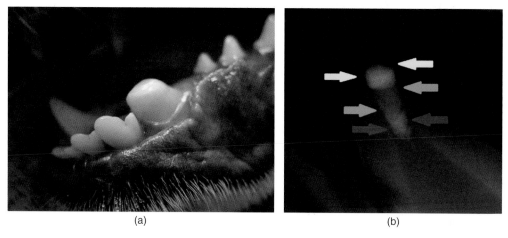

(a) (b)

Figure 7.12 Crown amputation and vital pulp therapy on a mandibular left canine (304). (a) Post-operative picture of the canine reduced approximately to the level of the incisors. (b) Post-operative intraoral dental radiograph revealing all three layers of a vital pulp therapy (VPT). Mineral trioxide aggregate (MTA) (red arrows); Glass ionomer (green arrows); Composite (yellow arrows). Source: Previously published in Veterinary Orthodontics with permission.

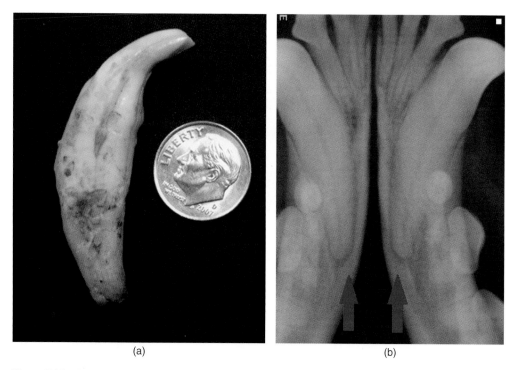

(a) (b)

Figure 7.13 Evidence showing why mandibular canine extractions are very challenging. (a) Mandibular canine tooth of a dog demonstrating the significant length of the root. (b) Dental radiograph of the mandibular canines in a small breed dog. The canines comprise the majority of the rostral jaw structure. Minimal bone apical to the roots of the canines (red arrows). The canine teeth are positioned lingually, especially nearer the apex. Source: Previously published in Veterinary Orthodontics and Dental Extractions Made Easier, with permission.

cause, research in human dentistry has demonstrated that retention of deciduous teeth is caused by an abnormal eruption path of the permanent tooth [32].

The high incidence of this condition in certain breeds makes genetics the most likely cause. In fact, there is an investigation into the genetic mutations which result in mesially displaced canine teeth in Shetland sheepdogs was performed at the University of Missouri. The purpose is to identify the gene(s) causing this condition in order to develop a DNA test to screen for this mutation and thus eliminate it from the breeding population [31]. Mesioversed canine teeth are strongly associated (88.2% of affected dogs) with X-linked hypohidrotic ectodermal dysplasia (XLHED) in dogs [33].

7.1.4.7 Clinical Appearance

Often this situation can occur either uni- or bilaterally. The maxillary canine tooth is displaced mesially, resulting in the long axis of the displaced canine tooth being more parallel to the hard palate and in contact with the 3rd incisor (Figure 7.14). The abnormal eruption path and contact with the third incisor typically creates infra-eruption of the canine tooth (Figure 7.15). The crowns of the maxillary canine teeth are also typically located mesial and often palatal to ipsilateral mandibular canine.

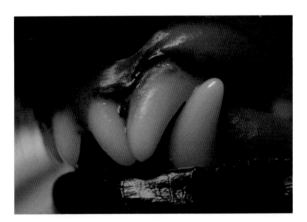

Figure 7.14 Intraoral dental picture of a 13-month-old Shetland Sheepdog with a mesioccluded left maxillary canine (204) [34] which is in contact with the ipsilateral third incisor (203) [35]. This has created crowding and infra-eruption of the tooth, both of which have resulted in the accumulation of plaque as well as foreign bodies. This in turn has led to the early onset of periodontal disease as demonstrated by the significant gingival inflammation.

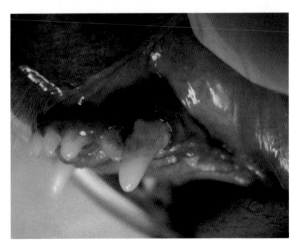

Figure 7.15 Intraoral dental picture of a 3-year-old Shetland Sheepdog with a mesioclused left maxillary canine. The malocclusion has resulted in infra-eruption of the tooth. Subsequently, early onset periodontal disease has occurred as demonstrated by the significant gingival inflammation and slight recession.

7.1.4.8 Sequelae

The crowding of the maxillary canine and third incisor tooth causes entrapment of food material and hastens plaque buildup compared to when a natural diastema is present between the teeth [36–42]. The infra-eruption results in a crown which is buried in the gingival/periodontal tissues. As gingiva cannot attach to enamel, a pseudopocket is created. This deep pocket is an environment with low oxygen tension, which promotes the growth of anaerobic bacterial pathogens commonly associated with periodontitis [36, 37, 43–45]. The combination of crowding with the third incisor and infra-eruption contributes to the early development of periodontal disease [30] (Figure 7.16).

The traumatic contact of the mesially displaced maxillary canine tooth with the ipsilateral mandibular canine can also cause labial displacement of the mandibular canine tooth (Figure 7.17). This may result in lip ulcers and oral pain as well as abnormal temperomandibular joint stress, concussive pulpitis associated pain, and possible pulp necrosis [46, 47].

Figure 7.16 Intraoral dental picture of a 16-month-old Shetland Sheepdog with a mesioclused left maxillary canine. Due to the infra-eruption (and crowding) there is already a 10-mm periodontal pocket on the mesial aspect of the tooth. Some of this (about 3-mm) is pseudopocketing from the infra-eruption, but the pocket is real and significant.

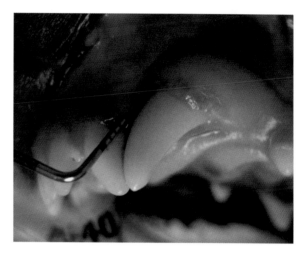

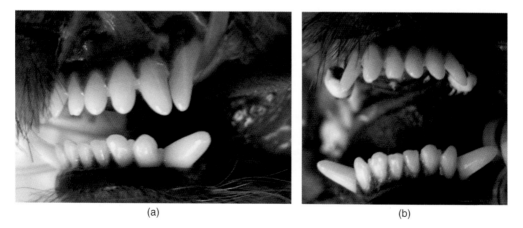

(a)   (b)

Figure 7.17 Intraoral dental pictures of a patient with mesiocclused maxillary canines which have caused the mandibular canines to be deflected buccally. (a) Left mesio-lateral view and (b) mesial view. This has created lip catching/trauma. Note that in (b) an orthodontic device has been applied to the maxillary canines.

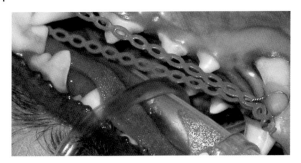

Figure 7.18 Maisel chain applied between the maxillary right canine and maxillary fourth premolar/mandibular first molar of a dog. Source: Image courtesy of Graham Thatcher and previously published in Veterinary Orthodontics, used with permission from Practical Veterinary Publishing.

7.1.4.9 Therapy

There are several options for management of mesioversed maxillary canine teeth [5, 30, 31]. These include extraction, coronal amputation and vital pulp therapy (or root canal treatment), and orthodontic movement of the tooth.

Orthodontic movement is the most correct (but also most challenging) method of correction. It is generally accomplished via the application of a Masel chain orthodontic appliance [46, 47] (Figure 7.18). Orthodontic movement of the mesioversed canine tooth requires a tipping force applied to the crown of the tooth, which moves the tooth around its center of rotation [15, 48]. The elastic is stretched between the crown of the canine tooth to be moved and the anchorage unit (which is typically the ipsilateral maxillary fourth premolar and first molar) [48].

This is a challenging procedure requiring several anesthetics and expertise in placement. Further, strict monitoring is necessary for optimal results. Care must be taken by the client not to allow the pet to damage the appliance. Finally, the mandibular canines can block the movement, requiring a "bite block" to temporarily keep the mouth open.

Extraction of the offending canine is the most common treatment for this condition since it can be performed by a general practitioner, and typically requires only one anesthesia. However, surgical extraction is very traumatic and it requires a mucoperiosteal flap and removal of bone as well as the loss of an important, potentially functional tooth [49]. Some of the risks of surgically extracting a maxillary canine tooth are wound dehiscence, hemorrhage, osteomyelitis, forcing of a root tip into the nasal cavity, jaw fracture, ocular damage, infection, and most commonly oronasal fistula formation [47, 49].

Extraction of the third incisor is a fairly straightforward therapy which can alleviate the crowding of the teeth and decrease periodontal disease. It does not solve the pseudopocket, but with consistent homecare and routine professional dental cleanings, periodontal health can often be maintained. However, an apically repositioned mucoperiosteal flap is the recommended therapy in cases of significant pseudopocketing to resolve this situation and create a normal gingival attachment [50] (see Figure 2.16 in Chapter 2). This is a one-step procedure that almost always results in a positive outcome, and therefore is this author's treatment of choice in most cases.

Coronal amputation of the mesioversed maxillary canine tooth with vital pulp therapy (or root canal treatment if the patient is mature), are both options available to save the mesioversed maxillary canine. These are treatments that can potentially prevent traumatic contact and/or crowding with the adjacent third maxillary incisor, however they do not provide the patient with a canine tooth in functional occlusion. This is generally not a recommended form of therapy; and this author tends to choose orthodontic movement or extraction of the canine or third incisor.

7.2 Gingival Enlargement

This condition was previously known as gingival hyperplasia, however hyperplasia is a histologic diagnosis and gingival enlargement (GE) is a clinical one. GE is a fairly common disease in dogs [51], and is defined as a proliferation of normal cellular components of the gingiva, especially the connective tissue [44]. It occurs most often in certain breeds, such as Collies and Mastiffs, but is by far the most common in Boxers, in which it may have a familial tendency [44, 52]. Gingival enlargement has a higher prevalence in males, possibly due to the presence of testosterone receptors within the gingiva [53]. It can also be caused by either acute or chronic inflammation of the gingiva [51]. Finally, it is known to be a drug reaction associated with several oral medications including immunosuppressants, anti-convulsants, angiotensin-converting-enzyme (ACE) inhibitors, cyclosporine, and calcium channel blockers [54–59].

Gingival enlargement is a benign lesion, but can have a similar appearance to neoplasia. There is a documented case where both benign gingival hyperplasia and malignant lesions were found in the same patient [60]. Therefore, any suspect gingival enlargements should be sampled and submitted for histopathologic evaluation. Additionally, dental radiographs should be made to evaluate the underlying bone prior to initiating the surgical procedure [61, 62].

With generalized gingival enlargement, the gingival tissue grows thicker and may cover part of or the entire crown (especially the mandibular incisors) (Figure 7.19). This overgrowth often creates pseudo-pockets which hinder plaque control (natural as well as homecare), resulting in increased plaque and calculus formation [44] (Figure 7.20). Consequently, gingival enlargement may result in early onset of periodontal disease [36, 37, 44, 45]. Therefore, it is important to remove the excess gingival tissue (gingivectomy) and restore normal physiological contours (gingivoplasty) [61, 63].

7.2.1 Treatment

If it is determined that the GE is being caused by a drug, ideally it is discontinued, which often will result in reversal of the enlargement. If it is not possible to change or stop the medication, or if GE has a genetic cause, excising the excess tissue (gingivectomy) is strongly recommended [64]. When performed early, it will decrease the amount of periodontal loss as well as make the procedure less invasive and shorter.

The standard gingivectomy technique is performed as follows [63] (Figure 7.21):

1. Measure the depth of the bottom of the pocket and mark with bleeding points (a).
2. Incise the gingiva at a 45° beveled angle (b).
3. Contour the excised gingiva and perform hemostasis (c).
4. The resultant gingiva has a beveled edge which decreases plaque attachment (d), but results in exposed edges which must heal by secondary intention (e).

The periodontal flap technique can also be used in certain cases (typically the mandibular cheek teeth) [64]. While more technical, this surgery will leave keratinized tissue facing out, decreasing pain and speeding return to function (Figure 7.22).

1. Perform a 70° *internal bevel* incision on all involved teeth (a).
2. Cut down along the tooth to remove epithelial attachment (b).

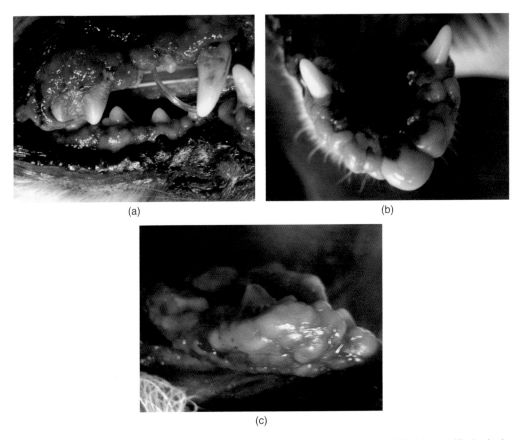

(a) (b)

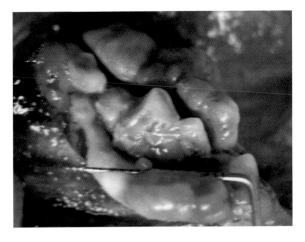

(c)

Figure 7.19 Marked gingival enlargement in a Boxer. Images showing the right side (a), mandibular incisor area (b), and right mandibular first molar (409) (c).

Figure 7.20 Intraoral dental picture of a Boxer with advanced gingival enlargement on the mandibular right first molar (409). The gingiva has been pulled back to reveal the significant calculus on the tooth due to lack of natural cleaning ability.

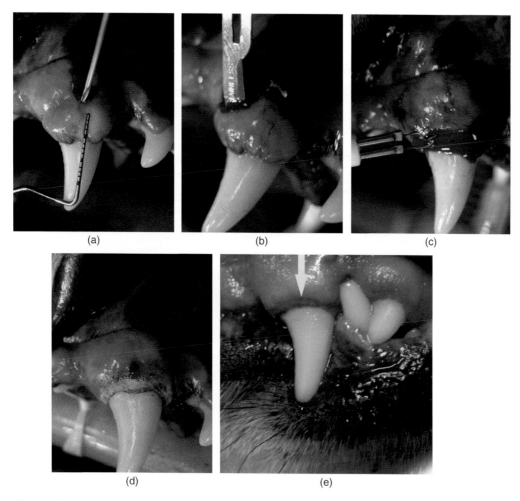

Figure 7.21 (a) Measure the depth of pocket and mark with bleeding points. (b) The gingiva is incised at a 45-degree angle. (c) The remaining gingiva is shaped. (d) Post-op picture. (e) 3-week recheck reveals slight continued inflammation. Standard gingivectomy technique. For further information on this technique see the chapter Gingival Surgery in the text Veterinary Periodontology.

3. Reflect the tissue to remain and remove the collar of extraneous tissue (c).
4. Close the incision with simple interrupted interdental incisions (d).
5. The surgical site heals faster via primary intention (e).

7.3 Chronic Ulcerative Paradental Stomatitis

While chronic ulcerative paradental stomatitis (CUPS) may be seen in any breed, it is most common in white, small breed dogs (especially Maltese) and Cavalier King Charles Spaniels [51]. CUPS is defined as an ulcerative, immune mediated reaction of the oral tissues, typically of the buccal mucosa.

Since these lesions consist histologically of lymphocytes and plasmacytes, CUPS represents an inflammatory rather than infectious etiology [65]. The antigen which stimulates the inflammatory

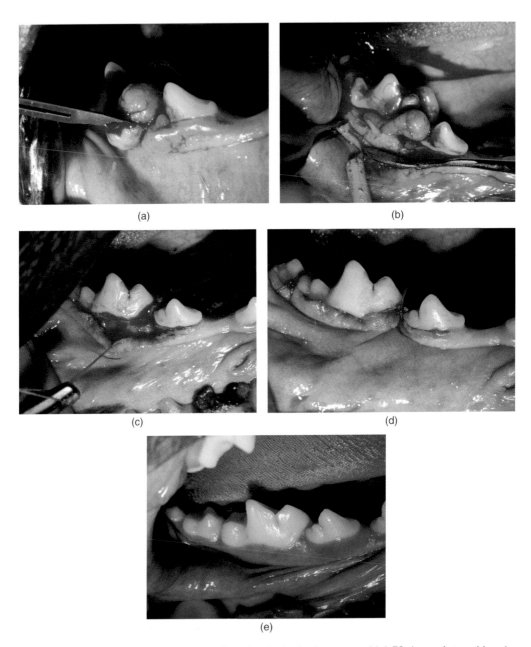

Figure 7.22 Periodontal flap surgery technique for gingival enlargement. (a) A 70-degree internal bevel incision is created on all involved teeth. (b) The epithelial attachment is released. (c) The tissue to remain is reflected and the collar of extraneous tissue removed. (d) The flaps are opposed and closed with simple interrupted interdental incisions. (e) 2-week recheck reveals complete healing and no inflammation.

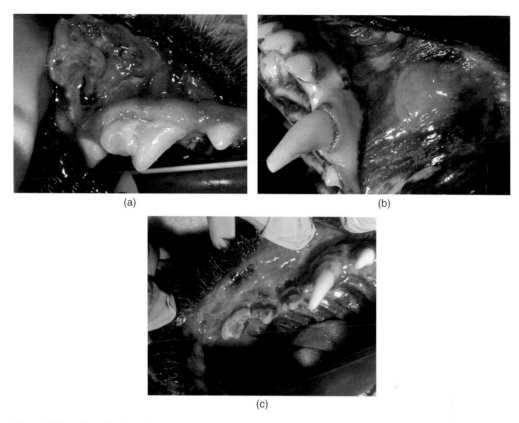

(a)   (b)

(c)

Figure 7.23 Chronic ulcerative paradental stomatitis. The buccal mucosa is severely ulcerated where it touches the teeth. (a) Maxillary right fourth premolar (108). (b) Maxillary left canine (204). (c) Severe case where not only the entire buccal mucosa, but also the attached gingiva is affected, and the inflammation is extending onto the palatine tissues.

reaction is presumed to be bacterial plaque [66]. In simple terms, this is appears to be an allergic reaction to the antigens present in plaque bacteria [67].

The presenting signs typically include: intense oral pain, halitosis, and partial to complete anorexia [67]. Conscious oral examination is often quite challenging due to patient pain. Examination under general anesthesia typically reveals significant dental plaque and calculus (unless the teeth were recently cleaned). In addition, gingivitis and often gingival recession or other signs of periodontal disease will commonly be seen.

The classic clinical sign is ulceration (often significant) of the buccal mucosa where it contacts the dentition (which is colloquially called a "kissing lesion") [67] (Figure 7.23). The lesions generally first occur (and are most significant over) the maxillary canine and carnassial teeth [65]. In addition, they tend to be worst in areas of gingival recession. In chronic/severe cases, the entire buccal mucosa and occasionally the lateral edges of the tongue may become involved (Figure 7.24). There is often a white, loose, and creamy discharge on the teeth (Figure 7.25). Finally, it is common to see an intertrigo affecting the mandibular lip (generally in the area of the frenulum or any skin folds) [67] (Figure 7.26). This may be due to pseudoptyalism (as the pet will avoid swallowing due to the pain). In chronic cases, scarring of the buccal mucosa may occur. Finally, osteomyelitis has been reported in association with CUPS [68].

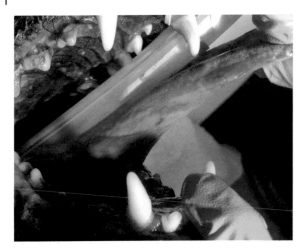

Figure 7.24 Ulceration of the lateral aspect of the tongue where it contacts the lingual surface of the mandibular teeth. This is only generally seen in severe cases. Homecare is rarely successful in these cases due to the difficulty in accessing this area. Early extractions are recommended.

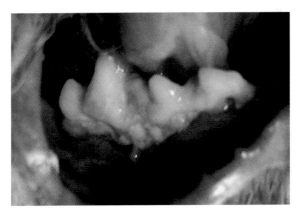

Figure 7.25 Loose creamy exudate on the teeth is quite common in CUPS cases.

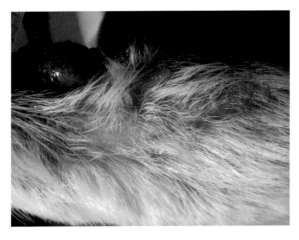

Figure 7.26 Intertrigo of the mandibular lip folds is very common in CUPS cases, and may persist eventhough the oral inflammation has resolved.

Prior to anesthesia, a complete physical examination and pre-anesthetic work-up should be performed. This would minimally include a complete blood panel and urinalysis to rule out systemic disease. CUPS patients typically have an elevated total protein, (polyclonal) hyperglobulinemia, and possibly a mild neutrophilia [65]. Other preanesthetic tests should be added based on these test results, as well as the patient's signalment.

Clinical signs are classic; however, histopathology should be performed to support the clinical diagnosis [69]. It will be consistent with significant ulcerative inflammation [69]. Bacterial and fungal cultures are generally mixed and unrewarding. Dental radiographs should be exposed to evaluate periodontal status [62]. The diagnosis is confirmed by a short-lived (a few weeks to months) positive response to a professional dental cleaning [67].

7.3.1 Treatment

The key to managing this disease process is strict plaque control [65, 67]. This is best achieved by a combination of a strict homecare regimen, regular dental cleanings, and selective to full mouth extractions. Tooth brushing and antiseptic rinses are the most effective means of plaque control [70]. A dental diet or effective chew can be used in addition to brushing and/or rinsing, or in cases of owner noncompliance [70]. It should be noted that without strict homecare this form of therapy will fail. Finally, a barrier sealant[1] has worked well in this author's hands in these cases when used consistently (see periodontal therapy above).

An important point to consider is that in the majority of cases, only a partial response should be expected, even with the strictest of homecare [67]. Resolution of most or all of the clinical signs may occur due to the stoic nature of dogs, however there is generally some degree of continued inflammation (and pain). These cases only achieve complete resolution with partial to full mouth extractions.

During the first anesthetic event, a professional dental cleaning should be performed. In addition, all periodontally diseased teeth (especially those with gingival recession) should be extracted [67]. Finally, histopathology +/− culture specimens should be obtained and submitted to a reference laboratory [69].

After the diagnosis is confirmed, council the owner for the need of long-term and consistent homecare which is required. In addition, regular (several times a year) cleanings are typically necessary. Patients with mild cases can often be treated in this manner.

If the regular cleanings and or homecare are not possible, the maxillary canine and carnassial (as well as any other teeth associated with buccal inflammation) should be extracted. Due to the difficulty in performing homecare, full mouth extractions are not unusual in these cases [51]. This form of therapy, while extreme, is curative in the vast majority of cases [32, 67] (Figure 7.27). When

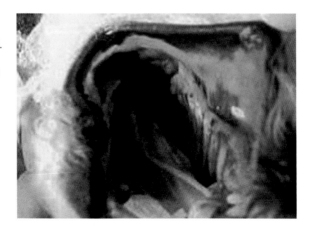

Figure 7.27 2-month recheck photo of the right side of a patient who received ½ mouth extractions for a severe case of CUPS. The patient is 100% healed and is acting much better than pre-operative. The patient is having the left side extracted today.

---

1 Oravet™ BI Deluth.

full mouth extractions are performed, it is not uncommon for clients to report that their dog "is acting like a puppy again."

Medical therapy has been unrewarding in this authors hands, however there are anecdotal reports from other dentists of successful therapy. One regimen which has minimal side effects consists of: pentoxifylline 20 mg/kg po bid, doxycycline 5 mg/kg po bid, and niacinamide 200–250 mg po bid. The other is cyclosporine and metronidazole at labeled dosages. If the latter medications are selected, clients must be informed prior to initiation of therapy and at regular intervals through the course of treatment of the side effects and long-term complications that can result from the long-term use of immunosuppressant drugs. Finally, regular blood and urine testing must be performed to ensure that untoward effects are not occurring. These factors, the involved costs, and the need for homecare must be weighed against surgical therapy, which is almost always curative.

7.4 Tight Lip Syndrome

This is a genetic condition which is seen mostly in the Shar-Pei breed [45, 51]. The classic appearance is where the rostral mandibular lip is very tight, leading to a shrinking of the mandibular vestibule. This often results in the lip being pulled over the mandibular incisors and in severe cases the canines [32] (Figure 7.28). The lip may be significantly affected, resulting in significant pain and even difficulty masticating. This condition may also result in disto-occlusion of the mandibular incisors and canines [32, 71].In severe cases, the lip may restrict mandibular growth and result in a mandibular brachygnathism (class II MAL) [9, 45] (Figure 7.29).

7.4.1 Therapy

Surgical correction (*vestibuloplasty*) is the treatment of choice for this condition [32, 51, 71–73]. This technique releases the tension on the jaw and teeth as well as normalizes the rostral mandibular vestibule. Surgery is initiated by incising the gingiva just apical to the mucogingival junction of the mandibular incisors and canines [45]. This incision should be made from frenulum to frenulum,

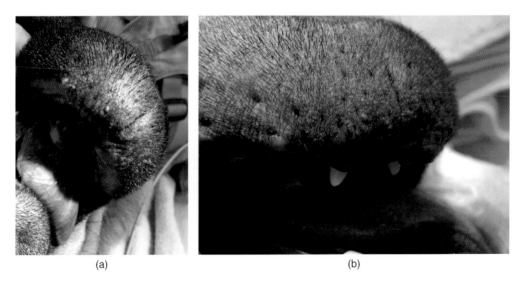

(a)   (b)

Figure 7.28 (a & b) A significant case of tight lip in a Shar Pei where the gums are overgrowing the incisors and canines.

Figure 7.29 The tight lip has resulted in a class II MAL.

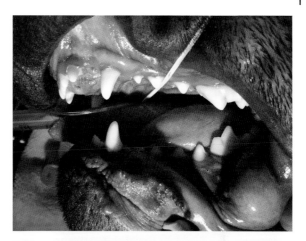

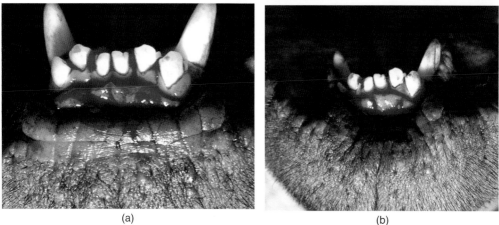

(a) (b)

Figure 7.30 (a & b) Post-operative picture of the vestibulopathy procedure performed on the patient in Figures 7.28 and 7.29.

exposing the entire rostral mandible to the level of the second premolars [45]. Following this, sharp/blunt dissection of the soft tissue and muscular attachments of the rostral mandibular lip is performed, resulting in the lip hanging down into the natural position. The flap is then left to heal by secondary intention, thus re-establishing normal lip position (Figure 7.30). Depending on the surgeon the area may be left open without sutures [9], sutured apically leaving the area exposed, or a spacer (such as a cut out piece of a rubber glove [51] or a graft harvested of buccal mucosa [73]) may be placed in the defect.

7.5 Craniomandibular Osteopathy

Craniomandibular osteopathy (CMO) is a proliferative bone disease seen in young dogs (4–8 months of age) [74]. It is most common in the West Highland white terrier, with a suspected autosomal recessive inheritance pattern [75, 76]. Other terrier breeds such as the Cairn and Scottish terriers are also overrepresented. It also has a genetic inheritance in Deutsch Drahthaar dogs [77].

CMO results from irregular and bilateral new bone formation typically involving the mandible (especially caudal body and rami), tympanic bulla, occipital bones, and the zygomatic portions of

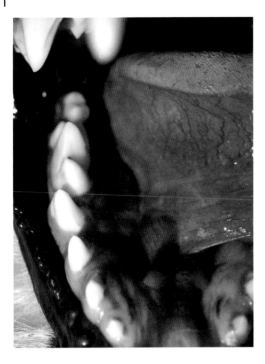

Figure 7.31 Intraoral dental radiograph of the right mandible of a dog with CMO. Note the mandibular swelling.

the temporal bone [78, 79]. It is neither inflammatory nor neoplastic in nature. The osseous lesions are the result of numerous complex changes in the growth and development of the bones in the area. The pathologic discrepancies include [74, 78]:

- osteoclastic resorption of lamellar bone
- replacement of lamellar bone by primitive coarse bone
- loss of normal bone marrow spaces
- replacement of marrow by a highly vascular fibrous stroma
- formation of new coarse trabecular bone with a pattern of irregular cement lines indicating the sporadic and rapid deposition and resorption of the abnormal bone.

The bony proliferation ends with skeletal maturation (e.g. when endochondral ossification ends at approximately 9–11 months of age) [74, 78]. At that time, the proliferative bone may regress to some extent. However, in the most severe cases the patient may be unable to open their mouth (see below) [78].

Clinical presentation includes [74]:

- thickening of the mandibular rami (Figure 7.31)
- mandibular pain
- difficulty or inability to open the mouth
- struggle in eating
- fever.

Furthermore, there are phases of acute disease (where the patient typically is painful) and remission [80]. In severely affected cases, jaw movement may be inhibited and atrophy of muscles of mastication may occur. Especially in larger dogs, mandibular swelling without pain or difficulty eating may occur. Finally, there appears to be a correlation between CMO and chronic otitis externa in West Highland White Terriers [76, 81].

Figure 7.32 Lateral skull film of a dog with CMO. The significant periosteal resection of the ventral aspect of the mandible is classic for this disease process.

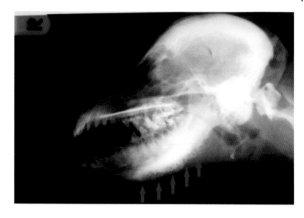

In the most severe cases, the angular process and enlarging tympanic bulla can fuse. This results in essentially a solid bar of abnormal bone resulting in a bone–bone connection [78]. Some terrier patients may also suffer from long bone or joint lesions resembling later stages of metaphyseal osteopathy [78, 79, 82].

Diagnosis is via a combination of radiographic and clinical signs. Radiographic changes are typically bilateral albeit asymmetric, with irregular bony proliferation involving both the mandible and temporomandibular joint (TMJ) about half the time [74, 80, 83] (Figure 7.32). Changes may be confined to the mandible or rarely only to the tympanic bulla/petrous temporal region. The tentorium ossium and calvarium are generally thickened along with the rest of the bones of the skull [80].

While not necessary in most cases, MRI has been shown to be an effective imaging option for CMO [84]. In atypical cases, biopsy of the affected bone may be recommended. The histology demonstrates resorption of the existing lamellae along with proliferation of coarse trabecular bone past normal periosteal boundaries. In addition, replacement of bone marrow by vascular fibrous stroma may be seen, as well as inflammatory cells involving the periphery of new bone. Finally, Irregular cement lines may be seen in the new/irregular bone [78, 80].

7.5.1 Therapy

Treatment with anti-inflammatories may temporarily reduce the pain, but whether it affects the growth of the lesions is unknown at this time. CMO is self-limiting, as the abnormal bone proliferation slows to a stop by around a year of age (following physeal closure) [79, 80]. Lesions may completely or partially regress at that time. However, significantly affected patients may still have difficulty in prehension and mastication [74, 85]. The prognosis is guarded when extensive changes affect the tympanic–petrous temporal areas and adjacent mandible. Ankylosis and adhesions may then develop, permanently restricting jaw movements and eating. Rostral mandibulectomy can be a useful salvage procedure in these cases [79]. Surgical excision of the bony lesions in these cases is typically unrewarding, occasionally leading to euthanasia [74].

7.6 Histologically Low-Grade, Biologically High-Grade, Fibrosarcoma

This is a unique oral tumor seen in large breed dogs, with golden retrievers being significantly overrepresented [86]. They represent a subset of traditional fibrosarcoma. They behave very aggressively biologically with quick expansion and bony invasion [34]. In addition, they appear to have a

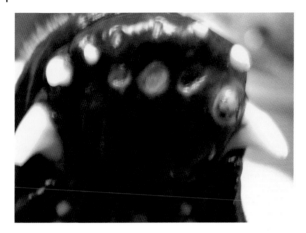

Figure 7.33 Intraoral dental picture of a 10-year-old golden retriever with a histologically low grade- biologically high grade fibrosarcoma of the rostral mandible. Note that the mass has normal overlying tissue. There is trauma from the maxillary incisors.

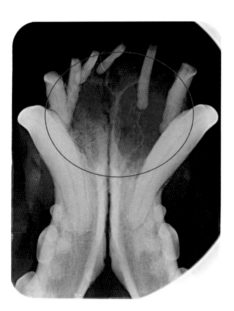

Figure 7.34 Intraoral dental radiograph of the area in (Figure 7.33) confirming the severe bony destruction typical of these lesions.

higher metastatic rate when compared to typical fibrosarcomas [34]. However, they tend to have an intact layer of epithelial tissue overlying the tumor, as opposed to the more ulcerative appearance of typical fibrosarcomas [87] (Figure 7.33). Most interestingly, they have a very benign appearance histologically, resembling gingival hyperplasia or inflammation [35, 87]. Knowledge of this possibility is important to avoid a treatment delay due to the benign pathology report [34].

Dental radiographs are a very important diagnostic tool in these cases. This is because it will provide evidence of the aggressive nature of this lesion, which will aid the pathologist and practitioner come to the correct diagnosis [62, 88] (Figure 7.34). Once the diagnosis is confirmed, staging as well as advanced imaging (computed tomography [CT]) should be performed for treatment planning.

The correct/ideal form of therapy for this tumor has not been determined. Different treatment modalities including surgical excision and/or radiation therapy (+/− hyperthermia) may increase survival times [35]. However, in general, prognosis is poor with a 12–16 month survival time with aggressive treatment [34].

References

1 Ulbricht, R.D. and Maretta, S.M. (2005). Orthodontic treatment using a direct acrylic inclined plane. *J. Vet. Dent.* 22 (1): 60–65.

2 Hale, F.A. (1996). Orthodontic correction of Lingually displaced canine teeth in a young dog using light-cured acrylic resin. *J. Vet. Dent.* 13 (2): 69–73.

3 Bannon, K. and Baker, L. (2008). Veterinary dentist at work: cast metal bilateral telescoping inclined plane for malocclusion in a dog. *J. Vet. Dent.* 25 (4): 250–258.

4 Oakes, A.B. and Beard, G.B. (1992). Lingually displaced mandibular canine teeth, orthodontic treatment alternatives in the dog. *J. Vet. Dent.* 9 (1): 20–25.

5 Lobprise, H.B. (2019). Occlusion and othodontics. In: *Wiggs' Veterinary Dentistry Principals and Practice*, 2e (eds. H.B. Lobprise and J.R. Dodd), 411–437. Hoboken: Wiley Blackwell.

6 Niemiec, B.A. (2010). Pathology in the Pediatric patient. In: *Small Animal Dental, Oral and Maxillofacial Disease a Color Handbook* (ed. B.A. Niemiec), 90–126. London: Manson Publishing Ltd.

7 Martel, D. (2013). Correction of Linguoclused mandibular canines. In: *Veterinary Orthodontics* (ed. B.A. Niemiec), 81–98. San Diego: Practical Veterinary Publishing.

8 Lewis, J.R. and Reiter, A.M. (2010). Anatomy and physiology. In: *Small Animal Dental, Oral and Maxillofacial Disease* (ed. B.A. Niemiec), 9–38. Boca Raton: CRC Press, Taylor & Francis Group.

9 Shipp, A.D. and Fahrenkrug, P. (1992). *Practitioner's Guide to Veterinary Dentistry*. Beverly Hills: Dr Shipps Laboratories.

10 Wiggs, R.B. and Loprise, H.B. (1997). Pedodontics. In: *Veterinary Dentistry-Principles and Practice* (eds. R.B. Wiggs and H.B. Loprise), 167–185. Philadelphia: Lippincott_Raven.

11 Wiggs, R.B. and Loprise, H.B. (1997). Oral anatomy and physiology. In: *Veterinary Dentistry-Principles and Practice* (eds. R.B. Wiggs and H.B. Loprise), 55–86. Philadelphia: Lippincott-Raven.

12 Carmichael, D. (1994). Crown amputation and vital Pulpotomy in a deciduous tooth. *Proc. World Vet. Dent. Cong.* 140.

13 Amimoto, A., Iwamoto, S., Taura, Y. et al. (1993). Effects of surgical orthodontic treatment for malalignment due to the prolonged retention of deciduous canines in young dogs. *J. Vet. Med. Sci.* 55 (1): 73–79.

14 Vandenbergh, L. (1993). The use of a modified quad-helix appliance in the correction of lingually displaced mandibular canine teeth in the dog. *J. Vet. Dent.* 10 (3): 20–25.

15 Surgeon, T.W. (2005). Fundamentals of small animal orthodontics. *Vet. Clin. North Am. Small Anim. Pract.* 35 (4): 869–889.

16 Verhaert, L. (1999). A removable orthodontic device for the treatment of lingually displaced mandibular canine teeth in young dogs. *J. Vet. Dent.* 16 (2): 69–75.

17 Holmstrom, S.E., Frost-Fitch, P., and Eisner, E. (2004). Orthodontics. In: *Veterinary Dental Techniques for the Small Animal Practitioner*, 3e (eds. S.E. Holmstrom, P. Frost-Fitch and E. Eisner), 499–558. Philadelphia: Elsevier.

18 Smith, M.M. (2013). Gingivectomy, gingivoplasty, and osteoplasty for mandibular canine tooth malocclusion. *J. Vet. Dent.* 30 (3): 184–197.

19 Carmichael, D. (2006). Canine orthodontics: providing healthy occlusions. *Vet. Med.*: 427–433.

20 Wiggs, R.B. and Loprise, H.B. (1997). Basics of orthodontics. In: *Veterinary Dentistry-Principles and Practice* (eds. R.B. Wiggs and H.B. Loprise), 435–481. Philadelphia: Lippincott-Raven.

21 Poeta, P., Igrejas, G., Gonçalves, A. et al. (2009). Influence of Oral hygiene in patients with fixed appliances in the Oral carriage of antimicrobial-resistant *Escherichia coli* and enterococcus isolates. *Oral Surg. Oral Med. Oral Pathol. Oral Radiol. Endod.* 108 (4): 557–564.

22 Furman, R. and Niemiec, B. (2013). Variation in acrylic inclined plane application. *J. Vet. Dent.* 30 (3): 161–166.

23 Pavlica, P. and Cestnik, V. (1995). Management of lingually displaced mandibular canine teeth in five bull terrier dogs. *J. Vet. Dent.* 12 (4): 127–129.

24 Moore, J. (2011). Vital pulp therapy. In: *Veterinary Endodontics* (ed. B.A. Niemiec), 78–92. San Diego: Practical Veterinary Publishing.

25 Niemiec, B.A. (2001). Assessment of vital pulp therapy for nine complicated crown fractures and fifty-four crown reductions in dogs and cats. *J. Vet. Dent.* 18 (3): 122–125.

26 Stoli, S. (2013). Class II malocclusions. In: *Veterinary Orthodontics* (ed. B.A. Niemiec), 99–109. San Diego: Practical Veterinary Publishing.

27 Niemiec, B.A. (2014). *Dental Extractions Made Easier* (ed. B.A. Niemiec). San Diego: Practical Veterinary Publishing.

28 Niemiec, B.A. (2008). Case based dental radiology. *Top. Compan. Anim. Med.* 24 (1): 4–19.

29 Mulligan, T., Aller, S., and Williams, C. (1998). *Atlas of Canine and Feline Dental Radiography*, 176–183. Trenton, NJ: Veterinary Learning Systems.

30 Niemiec, B.A. (2010). Problems with the pediatric patient. In: *Small Animal Dental, Oral & Maxillofacial Disease: A Color Handbook* (ed. B.A. Niemiec). London, UK: Manson Publishing.

31 Thatcher, G. (2013). Mesioclused maxillary canines. In: *Veterinary Orthodontics* (ed. B.A. Niemiec), 73–80. Tustin: Practical Veterinary Publishing.

32 Harvey, C.E. and Emily, P.P. (1993). *Small Animal Dentistry*. St. Louis: Mosby.

33 Lewis, J.R., Reiter, A.M., Mauldin, E.A., and Casal, M.L. (2010). Dental abnormalities associated with X-linked hypohidrotic ectodermal dysplasia in dogs. *Orthod. Craniofac. Res.* 13 (1): 40–47.

34 McEntee, M.C. (2012). Clinical behavior of nonodontogenic tumors. In: *Oral and Maxillofacial Surgery in Dogs and Cats* (eds. F.J.M. Verstraete and M. Lommner), 387–402. Philadelphia: Elsevier.

35 Dhaliwal, R.S. (2010). Malignant oral neoplasia. In: *Small Animal Dental, Oral and Maxillofacial Disease a Color Handbook* (ed. B.A. Niemiec), 225–235. London: Manson Publishing Ltd.

36 Wetering, A.V. (2011). Dental and oral cavity. In: *Small Animal Pediatrics* (eds. M.E. Peterson and M.A. Kutzler), 340–348. St. Louis, MO: Elsevier.

37 Hale, F.A. (2005). Juvenile veterinary dentistry. *Vet. Clin. Small Anim.* 35: 789–817.

38 Debowes, L.J. (2010). Problems with the gingiva. In: *Small Animal Dental, Oral and Maxillofacial Disease, a Color Handbook* (ed. B.A. Niemiec), 159–181. London: Manson.

39 Buckley, L.A. (1972). The relationship between malocclusion and periodontal disease. *J. Periodontol.* 43 (417): 415–417.

40 Startup, S. (2013). Rotated, crowded, and supernummery teeth. In: *Veterinary Orthodontics* (ed. B.A. Niemiec), 66–72. Tustin: Practical Veterinary Publishing.

41 Tondelli, P.M. (2019). Orthodontic treatment as an adjunct to periodontal therapy. *Dental Press J. Orthod.* 24 (4): 80–92.

42 Alsulaiman, A.A., Kaye, E., Jones, J. et al. (2018). Incisor malalignment and the risk of periodontal disease progression. *Am. J. Orthod. Dentofac. Orthop.* 153 (4): 512–522.

43 Newman, M.G., Takei, M., Klokkevold, P.R., and Carranza, F.A. (2011). *Carranza's Clinical Periodontology*, 11e. Philadelphia: Elsevier.

44 DeBowes, L. (2008). Problems with the gingiva. In: *A Colour Handbook of Small Animal Oral and Maxillofacial Diseases* (ed. B.A. Niemiec), 166–194. London, UK: Manson Publishing.

45 Niemiec, B.A. (2010). The importance of dental radiography. In: *Pathology in the Pediatric Patient* (ed. B.A. Niemiec), 89–126. London: Manson.

46 Gengler, W.R. (2004). Masel chain appliance for orthodontic treatment. *J. Vet. Dent.* 21 (4): 258–261.

47 Legendre, L. and Stepaniuk, K. (2008, 2008). Correction of maxillary canine tooth mesioversion in dogs. *J. Vet. Dent.* 25 (3): 216–221.

48 Theuns, P. (2013). Orthodontic tooth movement. In: *Veterinary Orthodontics* (ed. B.A. Niemiec), 22–35. Tustin: Practical Veterinary Publishing.

49 Niemiec, B.A. (2013). *Dental Extractions Made Easier*. Tustin, CA: Practical Veterinary Publishing.

50 Niemiec, B.A. (2013). Periodontal flap surgery. In: *Veterinary Periodontology* (ed. B.A. Niemiec), 206–248. Ames: Wiley Blackwell.

51 Wiggs, R.B. and Lobprise, H.B. (1997). *Veterinary Dentistry Principles & Practice*, 116. Philadelphia: Lippincott-Raven.

52 Burstone, M.S., Bond, E., and Litt, C.R. (1952). Familial gingival hypertrophy in the dog(boxer breed). *AMA Arch. Pathol.* 54 (2): 208–212.

53 Davan, D., Kozlovsky, A., Tal, H. et al. (1998). Castration prevents channel blocker-induced gingival hyperplasia in beagle dogs. *Hum. Exp. Toxicol.* 17 (7): 396–402.

54 Lafzi, A., Farahani, R.M., and Shoja, M.A. (2007). Phenobarbitol-induced gingival hyperplasia. *J. Contemp. Dent. Pract.* 8 (6): 50–56.

55 Eggerath, J., English, H., and Leichter, J.W. (2005). Drug-associated gingival enlargement: case report and review of aetiology, management and evidence-based outcomes of treatment. *J. N.Z. Soc. Periodontal.* 88: 7–14.

56 Nam, H.S., McAnulty, J.F., Kwak, H. et al. (2008). Gingival overgrowth in dogs associate with clinically relevant cyclosporine blood levels: observations in a canine renal transplantation model. *Vet. Surg.* 37 (3): 247–253.

57 Nishikawa, S., Nagata, T., Morisaki, I. et al. (1996). Pathogenesis of drug-induced gingival overgrowth. A review of studies in the rat model. *J. Periodontol.* 67 (5): 463–471.

58 Namikawa, K., Maruo, T., Honda, M. et al. (2012). Gingival overgrowth in a dog that received long-term cyclosporine for immune-mediated hemolytic anemia. *Can. Vet. J.* 53 (1): 67–70.

59 Pariser, M.S. and Berdoulay, P. (2011). Amlodipine-induced gingival hyperplasia in a Great Dane. *J. Am. Anim. Hosp. Assoc.* 47 (5): 375–376.

60 Sitzman, C. (2000). Simultaneous hyperplasia, metaplasia, and neoplasia in an 8 year-old boxer dog: a case report. *J. Vet. Dent.* 17 (1): 27–30.

61 Camargo, P.M. et al. (2006). Treatment of gingival enlargement. In: *Carranza's Clinical Periodontology*, 10e (eds. M.G. Newman et al.), 918–925. Philadelphia: Saunders.

62 Niemiec, B.A. (2011). The importance of dental radiology. *Eur. J. Comp. Anim. Pract.* 20 (3): 219–229.

63 Force, J. and Niemiec, B. (2009). Gingivectomy and gingivoplasty for gingival enlargement. *J. Vet. Dent.* 26 (2): 132–137.

64 Niemiec, B.A. (2013). Gingival surgery. In: *Veterinary Periodontology* (ed. B.A. Niemiec), 193–205. Ames: Wiley Blackwell.

65 Carmichael, D.T. (2004). Diagnosing and treating chronic ulcerative paradental stomatitis. *Vet. Med.* 99 (12): 1008–1011.

66 Smith, M.M. (1995). Oral and salivary gland disorders. In: *Textbook of Veterinary Internal Medicine*, 4e (eds. S.J. Ettinger and E.C. Feldman). Elsevier. PP 408–421.

67 Niemiec, B.A. (2008). Problems with the oral mucosa. In: *A Colour Handbook of Small Animal Oral and Maxillofacial Diseases* (ed. B.A. Niemiec), 183–198. London, UK: Manson Publishing.

68 Boutoille, F. and Hennet, P. (2011). Maxillary osteomyelitis in two Scottish terrier dogs with chronic ulcerative paradental stomatitis. *J. Vet. Dent.* 28 (2): 96–100.

69 Anderson, J.G., Peralta, S., Kol, A. et al. (2017). Clinical and histopathologic characterization of canine chronic ulcerative stomatitis. *Vet. Pathol.* 54 (3): 511–519.

70 Niemiec, B.A. (2012). Home plaque control. In: *Veterinary Periodontology* (ed. B.A. Niemiec), 175–185. Ames: Wiles.

71 McCoy, D.E. (1997). Surgical management of the tight lip syndrome in the Shar-Pei dog. *J. Vet. Dent.* 14 (3): 95–96.

72 Eisner, E.R. (2008). Vestibule deepening procedure for tight lip syndrome in the Chinese Shar-pei dog. *J. Vet. Dent.* 25 (4): 284–289.

73 Bellows, J. (2004). Oral surgical equipment, materials, and techniques. In: *Small Animal Dental Equipment, Materials, and Techniques, a Primer* (ed. J. Bellows), 297–361. Blackwell.

74 Taney, K.G. and Smith, M.M. (2010). Problems with muscles, bones, and joints. In: *Small Animal Dental, Oral, and Maxillofacial Disease, a Color Handbook* (ed. B.A. Niemiec), 199–204. London: Manson.

75 Padget, G.A. and Mostosky, U.V. (1986). Animal model: the mode of inheritance of craniomandibular osteopathy in West Highland White terrier dogs. *Am. J. Med. Genet.* 25: 9.

76 Pratschke, K.M. (2019). Severe chronic otitis and craniomandibular osteopathy in West Highland white terriers. *J. Small Anim. Pract.* 60 (8): 519.

77 Vagt, J. and Distl, O. (2018). Complex segregation analysis of craniomandibular osteopathy in Deutsch Drahthaar dogs. *Vet. J.* 231: 30–32.

78 Riser, W.H. (1993). Canine craniomandibular osteopathy. In: *Disease Mechanisms in Small Animal Surgery* (ed. M.J. Bojrab), 892–899. Philadelphia: Lippincott Williams & Wilkins.

79 Johnson, K.A. and Watson, A.D.J. (2005). Skeletal diseases. In: *Textbook of Veterinary Internal Medicine*, 6e (eds. S.J. Ettinger and E.C. Feldman), 1976–1978. St. Louis: Elsevier.

80 Halliwell, W.H. (1993). Tumor-like lesions of bone. In: *Disease Mechanisms in Small Animal Surgery* (ed. M.J. Bojrab), 934–935. Philadelphia: Lippincott Williams & Wilkins.

81 Beever, L., Swinbourne, F., Priestnall, S.L. et al. (2019). Surgical management of chronic otitis secondary to craniomandibular osteopathy in three West Highland white terriers. *J. Small Anim. Pract.* 60 (4): 254–260.

82 Pettitt, R., Fox, R., Comerford, E.J., and Newitt, A. (2012). Bilateral angular carpal deformity in a dog with craniomandibular osteopathy. *Vet. Comp. Orthop. Traumatol.* 25 (2): 149–154.

83 Shorenstein, B., Schwartz, P., and Kross, P.H. (2014). What is your diagnosis? Craniomandibular osteopathy. *J. Am. Vet. Med. Assoc.* 245 (5): 491–492. https://doi.org/10.2460/javma.245.5.491.

84 Matiasovic, M., Caine, A., Scarpante, E., and Cherubini, G.B. (2016). Imaging diagnosis-magnetic resonance imaging features of craniomandibular osteopathy in an airedale terrier. *Vet. Radiol. Ultrasound.* 57 (3): E27–E29.

85 Montgomery, R. (2003). Miscellaneous orthopaedic diseases. In: *Textbook of Small Animal Surgery* (ed. D. Slatter), 2255. Philadelphia: WB Saunders.

86 Ciekot, P.A., Powers, B.E., Withrow, S.J. et al. (1994). Histologically low-grade, yet biologically high-grade, fibrosarcomas of the mandible and maxilla in dogs: 25 cases (1982–1991). *J. Am. Vet. Med. Assoc.* 204: 610–615.

87 Soukup, J. and Lewis, J. (2019). Oral and maxillofacial tumors, cyts, and tumor like lesions. In: *Wiggs' Veterinary Dentistry Principals and Practice*, 2e (eds. H.B. Lobprise and J.R. Dodd), 131–153. Hoboken: Wiley Blackwell.

88 Niemiec, B.A. The importance of and indications for dental radiology. In: *Practical Veterinary Dental Radiology* (eds. B.A. Niemiec, J. Gawor and V. Jekel), 5–30. CRC press.

8

Anesthetic Management of Toy and Small Breed Dogs
Amber Hopkins

VCA Alameda East Veterinary Hospital, Denver, CO, USA

8.1 Introduction

There are no actual studies that define the difference between small, toy and miniature breed dogs. Some base the title on height at the withers and others base it on their body weight. Generally, the term is used to describe a very small dog. For the purpose of this chapter, we will focus on what the American Kennel Club (AKC) describes as "x-small dogs" (Table 8.1).

   While very small breeds do pose some unique challenges to the anesthetist, there are no studies demonstrating a statistically significant increase or decrease in anesthetic risk in toy and small breeds. This chapter will focus on these unique challenges and provide guidance on how to mediate them.

8.2 Body Size

There are several potential challenges with toy and small breed dogs, which can make anesthesia more challenging. The most obvious is their actual size, which can pose many difficulties including catheterization, trauma during restraint, difficulty in maintaining normothermia, and difficultly in accessing and assessing them during a procedure.

8.2.1 Restraint and Catheterization

It is not uncommon for these patients to present with a higher degree of anxiety and aversion to handling, particularly of their legs and feet. This results in more stress for the client, staff, and obviously the patient, but also makes obtaining diagnostics (blood and urine samples as well as radiographs) and placing an intravenous catheter more difficult. These dogs also have smaller bones, which makes them more fragile. Finally, many of these patients have very small vessels making catheter placement even more difficult. Therefore, it is important that we consider measures that reduce patient anxiety and allow for easier and less aggressive handling.

   When appropriate, it can be quite beneficial to prescribe anti-anxiety medications, to be given before their transport into the hospital. Historically, oral acepromazine was often prescribed to patients to take before travel. Many clinicians report the effects of oral acepromazine to be unpredictable, resulting in either minimal or significant sedation with prolonged recoveries.

Breed Predispositions to Dental and Oral Disease in Dogs, First Edition. Edited by Brook A. Niemiec.
© 2021 John Wiley & Sons, Inc. Published 2021 by John Wiley & Sons, Inc.

Table 8.1 Breeds defined by the American Kennel Club as X-small breeds.

Affenpinscher	Miniature Pinscher
Biewer Terrier	Papillon
Bolognese	Pomeranian
Brussels Griffon	Poodle (Toy)
Chihuahua	Russian Toy
Chinese Crested	Russian Tsvetnaya
Japanese Chin	Silky Terrier
Maltese	Toy Fox Terrier
Manchester (Toy) Terrier	Yorkshire Terrier

Table 8.2 Common pre-anesthetic oral sedatives.

Drug	Class	Dose range canine	Dose range feline
Trazodone	SARI	3–7 mg kg^{-1} PO q12 h	1–2 mg kg^{-1} PO q12 h
Acepromazine	Phenothiazine	0.5–2.2 mg kg^{-1} PO q6–8 h	0.5–2.2 mg/kg PO
Lorazepam	Benzodiazepine	0.02–0.1 mg kg^{-1} PO q8–12 h	0.125–0.25 mg/cat
Gabapentin	Anticonvulsant	5–30 mg kg^{-1} PO q8–12 h	3–10 mg kg^{-1} PO q8–24 h

Source: Perrin et al. (2014) [35].

Additionally, because of its α-adrenergic and dopaminergic receptor antagonistic properties, vasodilation can occur which negatively affects thermoregulation and can create perioperative hypotension. This particular category of patients is also more prone to perioperative hypothermia due to their greater body surface area to mass ratio, making acepromazine's effects on vascular tone and thermoregulation of potential concern [1]. Though there are a variety of other anxiolytic medications for pre-anesthetic oral use to choose from (Table 8.2), trazodone has become a common and quite reliable choice for pre-anesthetic relief of anxiety. Trazodone is a serotonin receptor antagonist and reuptake inhibitor [1]. The anxiolytic properties of trazodone seem to be related to the receptor site activities of the drug, which alter serotonin and likely reduces aminobutyric acid concentrations in the cerebral cortex [2, 3]. There have been five studies in dogs highlighting its efficacy in reducing patient stress behaviors, noting it to be well-tolerated and safe as a single agent [4]. There have been concerns raised over the potential risk for serotonin syndrome, with the increasing number of patients receiving drugs that affect serotonin levels. This emphasizes the need for a thorough medical history. Clinically reported occurrences of serotonin syndrome in veterinary patients are uncommon, but as more patients are prescribed drugs such as selective serotonin reuptake inhibitors (SSRI), serotonin and norepinephrine reuptake inhibitors (SNRI), tricyclic antidepressants, monoamine oxidase inhibitors (MAOI) (e.g. tramadol, fluoxetine, selegiline, etc.) this could change [4]. More recently, the combination of some of the medications listed above with or without the addition of Melatonin has been advocated for pre-hospital visit administration.

Placement of an intravenous catheter can be potentially aversive to dogs. Easier catheter placement can be facilitated by two factors: premedication and reduction of discomfort. Premedication is provided for a variety of reasons including sedation, analgesia, easier and safer handling of patients, reduction in the amount of induction drug(s) needed, and minimum alveolar concentration (MAC) reduction. When possible, premedication can significantly reduce the patients' resistance to restraint and catheter placement. Sedation and the reduction of nociception are particularly beneficial for catheter placement. Beyond injectable analgesics, topical local anesthetics can be used to promote easier intravenous catheter placement. EMLA cream is a topical eutectic mixture of the local anesthetics, lidocaine, and prilocaine and has been demonstrated in humans, dogs, cats, and rabbits to desensitize the skin to make placement of an IV catheter less aversive to the patient [5–9]. EMLA cream application appears to be safe in laboratory animals, cats, and dogs, with the most significant side effect found to be blanching or reddening of the skin [6]. The only notable downside is the onset time. In order to achieve a significant decrease in response to catheter placement, the anesthetic cream needs to be applied directly to the skin at least 60 minutes prior to venipuncture [5].

8.2.2 Hypothermia

Hypothermia is one of the most common anesthetic complications in dogs and cats. Unfortunately, it is often the one that is the least proactively and aggressively managed by many veterinary professionals despite the vast number of complications it can create (Table 8.3). Hypothermia is classified into primary and secondary varieties. Primary hypothermia is generally associated with environmental exposure in patients with normal heat production and thermoregulatory control [10]. Anesthetic related hypothermia is classified as secondary hypothermia or hypothermia that occurs secondary to drug therapy that alters heat production, and/or the patient's thermoregulatory ability [10]. Anesthesia results in body temperature decline via many mechanisms including:

Table 8.3 Consequences of hypothermia.

Body system	Consequences
Cardiovascular	• Peripheral vasoconstriction and tachycardia • Bradycardia unresponsive to anticholinergics • Vasodilation and hypotension • Arrhythmias and conduction abnormalities
Respiratory	• Bronchospasm • Respiratory depression
Hepatic/gastrointestinal	• Reduced hepatic blood flow and metabolism • Decreased GI motility • Increased risk for poor GI perfusion, leading to GI ulceration • Decreased insulin production and hyperglycemia
Renal	• Cold diuresis and reduction in ADH leading to hypovolemia • Reduced renal blood flow and increased risk for acute kidney injury (AKI)
Cerebral/neuromuscular	• Shivering increasing oxygen consumption • Changes in cerebral electrical activity and temperature dependent brain function
Clinical pathology	• Inhibition of the clotting cascade • Impaired platelet function • Splenic/hepatic sequestration of platelets • Leukopenia leading to impaired wound healing • Electrolyte disturbances • Hypoglycemia

Source: Brodeur et al. (2017) [10].

Table 8.4 Mechanisms of heat loss.

Mechanism	Physiology	Examples	Solutions
Conduction	Transfer of heat from body to objects it is in contact with	Direct contact with a table colder than the patient	Lay patient on top of non-porous heated blanket
Convection	Transfer of heat from body to surrounding air	Low OR temperature, open body cavity	Warm forced air blankets
Radiation	Transfer of heat from body to objects it is NOT in contact with	Surrounding room equipment and OR with temperatures lower than patient	Warm forced air blankets
Evaporation	Loss of heat energy contained in water vapor	Use of cold surgical scrub/alcohol, wet fur, respiratory secretions, open wounds/cavity	Wrapping paws with non-porous wraps, warm inspired air, warm lavage

delivery of dry and cold inhalant gases, administration of cold IV fluids, open body cavities, laying on cold surfaces, peripheral vasodilation from inhalant or injectable drugs, and drug related changes to the thermoregulatory center in the brain.

Heat is lost by several mechanisms including convection, conduction, evaporation, and radiation (Table 8.4). It is, therefore, the anesthetist's obligation to minimize heat loss by addressing these mechanisms. Small and neonatal patients have a greater body surface area to mass ratio than larger patients, predisposing them to greater conductive, convective, and radiation heat loss through their skin and therefore hypothermia [11]. In many cases, depending on the procedure being performed, these patients can be harder to cover sufficiently with warming devices due to their small size. Fortunately, the ability to adequately cover dental patients is not generally as challenging as it is for other procedures. These patients can be more difficult to keep warm, however, as they are more prone to becoming soaked with fluid during dental scaling. In fact, water has high thermal conductivity, predisposing them to hypothermia [12]. Therefore, minimizing the amount of fur that is soaked with any fluid and ensuring that the patient is as dry as possible in the recovery period is of importance.

In humans, pre-warming has been shown to significantly decrease perioperative heat loss. The evidence in dogs as to the benefit or necessity of pre-warming is less convincing [13]. Passive warming (e.g. blankets, towels) alone is not as beneficial as warming patients, but can reduce heat loss by counteracting conductive and convective losses. Active warming should be conducted in any patient anesthetized for more than 20 minutes, especially in the smaller patients and in the recovery period if the patient is not normothermic at that time [13] (Figure 8.1). Forced air warming has been shown to be more efficacious than resistive polymer electric blankets [14–16]. The combination of passive warming prior to induction and active warming once the patient is anesthetized, however, is essential. Other methods for warming can include wrapping extremities with non-porous materials, fluid warmers, and circulating water blankets. One should take caution that just as these patients can become cold quickly, they can also rewarm very quickly and may overheat. These patients should have their temperatures monitored for a minimum of every 15 minutes and warming efforts adjusted accordingly.

Figure 8.1 Active warming of the smaller patient.

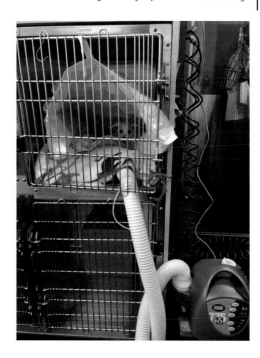

8.3 Congenital Predispositions

Prior to any anesthesia it is important to obtain a thorough history, including past anesthetic procedures, and perform a full physical exam. Small and toy breeds can have congenital abnormalities that can significantly change the potential anesthetic complications the patient is at risk for, what anesthetic drugs should be considered, and how the patient is monitored and managed during the peri-anesthetic period. Some form of pre-anesthetic blood work is recommended. The extensiveness of pre-anesthetic work-up depends on the age of the patient, history, intended procedure, and physical exam findings.

8.3.1 Portosystemic Shunts

Single congenital extrahepatic shunts are most commonly found in small breed dogs such as Yorkshire Terriers, Schnauzers, Maltese, Shih Tzus, and Pugs [17]. Though neurologic signs are most common, in some patients the only exhibited signs may be weight loss, vomiting, diarrhea, cystitis, or those related to urinary tract obstruction from urate calculi and ammonium biurate crystal formation. Routine pre-anesthetic blood work and urinalysis may show a microcytic anemia, hypoalbuminemia, hypoglycemia, decreased blood urea nitrogen (BUN), elevated liver enzymes and/or ammonium biurate urinary crystals [17]. Medical management should be started prior to any anesthetic procedure, if not already initialed. Levetiracetam 20 mg kg^{-1} PO q8h started at a minimum of 24 hours before anesthesia has been recommended to minimize the risk of seizures [18]. In these patients, the use of drugs that are minimally metabolized by the liver (e.g. propofol) and/or are reversible are preferred. If the use of drugs that rely highly on the liver for metabolism are indicated, their doses should be reduced. There are mixed opinions on the use of benzodiazepines in these patients. Flumazenil, the antagonist for benzodiazepines, had been shown to improve clinical signs of hepatic encephalopathy in some human patients. Several studies have been done in human patients since that time, to identify the etiology of this effect, but results have been inconsistent [19, 20]. Benzodiazepines are therefore a reasonable premedication or co-induction agent in patients with liver dysfunction and even potentially those with portosystemic shunts (PSS), though low doses should be used. In patients that have any evidence of severe liver dysfunction, evidence of cirrhosis or hepatic encephalopathy, use of benzodiazepines should be used with caution and if used, used at low doses and access to flumazenil is recommended. Generally, these patients do well during anesthesia; however, maintaining intra-operative perfusion, monitoring their glucose levels and closely assessing them in the recovery period for any seizure activity is important.

8.3.2 Tracheal Collapse

Tracheobronchomalacia, weakened tracheal cartilage causing dorsoventral flattening and laxity of the dorsal trachealis muscles, can lead to partial or complete tracheal collapse. It occurs most commonly in small and toy breeds, particularly Yorkshire Terriers, Pomeranians, Toy and Miniature Poodles, Chihuahuas, and some brachycephalic dogs [21]. History or physical exam may alert you to some of the common clinical signs including a "goose honk" cough, exercise intolerance, respiratory distress, and even cyanosis. Palpation of the ventrocervical region may elicit a cough further increasing suspicion. Most of the anesthetic risk in these patients is associated with the pre and post-anesthetic periods. Pre-operatively, the patient's stress level should be minimized, and sedation provided prior to IV catheter placement. The ideal endotracheal tube size would be one that does not require a lot of air for inflation of the cuff, but should also not be snug after placement, as to avoid tracheal irritation and coughing post-operatively. On recovery, the endotracheal tube should be removed when the patient is awake enough to lift its head and swallow, but before the patient begins coughing. These patients may need post-operative sedation if they become stressed to the point of obstruction of their airway and additional endotracheal tubes and induction agents should be at the ready in case reintubation is necessary.

8.3.3 Cardiac Disease

Toy and small breed dogs have been found to have a high incidence of cardiac disease, specifically myxomatous mitral valve disease. In fact, one study evaluating the cause of death in 74,556 canine patients, found that nearly 75% of breeds with average body weight of less than 9 kg were reported to have cardiovascular issues as a major cause of death compared to only 25% of breeds with average weights over 9 kg [22]. Though not specifically documented in the veterinary literature, in humans shorter height has also been linked to a higher incidence of cardiovascular disease [23] leading to the question of whether this is true in toy breed dogs as well. Cardiovascular disease can have a significant impact on a how a patient does during and after an anesthetic procedure, making pre-anesthetic physical exam and history of utmost importance. If upon cardiac auscultation, there is suspicion for an arrhythmia or a murmur is present, thoracic radiographs, ECG, and an echocardiogram should be recommended, to determine what disease process is present and how severe the disease is. Patients with cardiac disease can generally be safely anesthetized, but knowing what disease process is present and how significant it is can drastically change how that patient is managed.

8.4 Anesthetic and Procedural Challenges

8.4.1 Pre-anesthetic Phase

When developing an anesthetic protocol, there are no specific drug protocols for small and toy breeds, unless there are preexisting co-morbidities. What should be considered is the expected duration of the procedure and the anticipated level of post-procedure pain. Pre-medications should provide adequate sedation and analgesia, particularly if anything beyond a simple scaling is anticipated. One area that needs to be considered during the pre-medication period is the amount of volume being delivered if administration is intramuscular (IM). Primary IM injection sites include epaxial muscle, quadriceps, and triceps. Because these are smaller muscles in tiny patients, guidelines have been established as to the amount of volume per site that is considered to be in good practice, to avoid damage to tissues and minimize pain. For dogs, this volume has been determined to be 0.25 ml/kg/injection site [24]. In general, it is also recommended that no more than two sites be used whenever possible. On the other hand, for some highly concentrated drugs (e.g. ketamine, dexmedetomidine) dilution may be necessary to ensure more accurate dose administration, therefore one should always keep good practice volumes in mind.

8.4.2 Induction Phase

Prior to the induction of anesthesia, all necessary equipment should be at hand, all endotracheal tubes and the anesthesia machine leak tested, and all monitoring equipment checked for functionality. Choosing an appropriate breathing circuit comes with some varied opinions. There is currently no minimum patient size established for using a rebreathing system vs. a non-rebreathing system. Most would agree that any patient less than 2.5–3 kg should be maintained with a non-rebreathing circuit. This system minimizes mechanical dead space and resistance to breathing. Excessive mechanical dead space leads to rebreathing of carbon dioxide and decreases the effective tidal volume available for gas exchange. Common areas of mechanical dead space are: the patient end of breathing circuits; any endotracheal length beyond the tip of the patient's nose; side-stream capnograph adapters; in-line capnographs; and elbow adapters [34]. Those patients between 3 and 10 kg may be maintained on a pediatric rebreathing system so long as oxygenation and expired end-tidal carbon dioxide are monitored and maintained within normal limits.

Before intubation, the endotracheal tube should be measured for appropriate length. The beveled tip of the tube should lie at or just rostral to the thoracic inlet, while the end that attaches to the breathing circuit, should ideally not extend past the tip of the nose. Often in dental patients, the tube is left slightly longer to facilitate easier access and visualization of the oral cavity for the dental practitioner. One should remember that this increases dead space and should be minimized as much as possible, especially in smaller patients. Once the patient is intubated, the endotracheal tube cuff should be inflated in small increments, only to the point of eliminating the leak. The goal is to maintain an airtight seal without impeding blood flow through the tracheal mucosa. Airway pressures of 18–25 mm Hg have been recommended to provide safe airway occlusion [25–27]. Briganti et al. [28] evaluated four common methods for inflation of endotracheal tube cuffs and found that none consistently provided cuff pressures within the acceptable ranges. There are currently a few devices on the market to measure cuff pressure and minimize the risk of cuff over-inflation, but none have been proven to be accurate in both low pressure/high volume and high pressure/low volume endotracheal tubes and none to be superior to their competition of the publication date. One of the more devastating anesthetic complications in toy and small breed dogs, as well as cats, is over-inflation of the endotracheal (ET) tube cuff, resulting in tracheal wall inflammation, disruption of tracheal blood flow, resulting in post-anesthetic strictures or necrosis and tracheal rupture [25, 27]. This situation can result in significant complications and even death. Recommendations to minimize the risk of this complication include: proper cuff inflation using a pressure manometer; disconnecting the patient from the breathing circuit before rotating; and assuring that the patient is turned slowly and in a single plane. It is also important to note that several studies have demonstrated that cuff pressure significantly decreases throughout the procedure without intervention [26]. During dental procedures, there is a high likelihood of the oral cavity collecting significant amounts of water and debris, so it critical that the endotracheal cuff is checked frequently to minimize the risk of aspiration.

8.4.3 Maintenance Phase

Once the patient has been anesthetized, lubrication of the eyes should occur and be repeated every 30 minutes. It has been established that decreased tear production is a risk factor for corneal ulceration or erosion and that general anesthesia significantly decreases tear production [30]. It has also been established that lengthy procedures, lateral positioning, and procedures of the head all increase this risk [29]. Based on the variable residence time of ocular lubricants, dependent on their formulation and concentration, as well as the likelihood of chemical, debris, and physical contact of the cornea during dentistry procedures, it is recommended that eyes be lubricated every 30 minutes. It is also worth noting that tear production remains decreased for up to 24 hours post-anesthesia and consideration for eye lubrication during that time may be of benefit [30].

Fortunately for veterinary dental procedures, access to the patient is usually not inhibited. For other surgical procedures, these small patients may be under drapes and far from the anesthetist, making visual, and hands-on assessment difficult due to their small size. Pre-anesthetic planning is essential to assure best patient care. This means that prior to moving a patient into an operating room and prior to draping a patient, the anesthetist should assure the catheter is patent, that there is no reason to believe a second catheter will be needed and that monitoring equipment is on and functioning appropriately. You may also consider attaching mini extension sets and/or micro Y-sets ahead of time to allow prompt drug delivery when needed, and an extra port for delivery of any unexpected constant rate infusions (CRIs), minimizing the risk of volume overload with excessive flush.

Monitoring these patients can also be challenging. Though there are some devices designed specifically for veterinary patients, many common monitoring devices are designed for humans. These can sometimes be too large for small patients, slip off patients easily or occlude very tiny vessels requiring more hands-on manipulation. The size of the patient can also affect the accuracy of some non-invasive blood pressure monitors. Cuff size plays a significant role in the accuracy of non-invasive blood pressure (NIBP). If a blood pressure cuff is too large, as can occur in very small patients, the reading obtained can be falsely low. Unfortunately, there is little agreement as to the best NIBP monitoring device. Oscillometric devices have been shown to be inaccurate in smaller patients [30, 31]. Some have suggested that Doppler blood pressure measurement be used for patients less than 10 kg [32], while others have concluded that Doppler readings are in poor agreement with invasive measures and could be misleading [32].

8.4.4 Recovery Phase

It has been reported that over half of all anesthetic related deaths occur within the recovery period with over 50% of those occurring in the first three hours of recovery [33]. Due to the retrospective nature of the study, the underlying cause of these deaths were not definitively determined; however it is likely that several factors contribute. It is not uncommon for anesthetists (veterinarians or technicians) to be relieved when a patient is "awake" and can now move on to other duties or other patients. Once the patient is extubated, they may no longer have an assured and/or protected airway. They no longer have monitoring equipment attached to them and once extubated they are often left alone without much visual monitoring. If a patient wakes up poorly, they may be given additional pain medications or sedatives and once relaxed may be left alone without any real oversight. This can predispose them to hypoventilation, apnea, regurgitation, arrhythmias, or dramatic changes in cardiac output. This highlights the importance of diligent and continuous post-operative monitoring, particularly if these patients already have underlying cardiac or respiratory disease processes or if additional analgesics or sedatives were needed upon recovery. For all recovering patients, there should be active monitoring and vitals taken every 15–30 minutes for the 3 hours following extubation or until standing, to assure they are warming and recovering appropriately. If the patient has just received additional sedation medication, is very cold or is a high-risk patient, they should be evaluated more frequently.

8.5 Conclusion

While not at an increased risk per se, toy and small breed dogs can certainly have additional anesthetic challenges as compared to larger breeds. Minimizing their stress, appropriate pre-anesthetic screening and planning, maintenance of normothermia and diligent post-anesthetic monitoring are all vital in assuring the safest peri-anesthetic outcome possible.

References

1 Riviere, J.E., Papich, M.G., and Adams, H.R. (2018). *Veterinary Pharmacology and Therapeutics*, 10e. Wiley Blackwell.

2 Stahl, S.M. (2009). Mechanism of action of trazodone: a multifunctional drug. *CNS Spectr.* 14 (10): 536–546.

3 Luparini, M.R., Garrone, B., Pazzagli, M. et al. (2004). A cortical GABA-5HT interaction in the mechanism of action of the antidepressant trazodone. *Prog. Neuro-Psychopharmacol. Biol. Psychiatry* 28 (7): 1117–1127.

4 Sinn, L. (2018). Advances in behavioral psychopharmacology. *Vet. Clin. Small Anim.* 48 (3): 457–471.

5 van Oostrom, H. and Knowles, T.G. (2018). The clinical efficacy of EMLA cream for intravenous catheter placement in client-owned dogs. *Vet. Anaesth. Analg.* 45 (5): 604–608.

6 Flecknell, P.A., Liles, J.H., and Williamson, H.A. (1990). The use of lignocaine-prilocaine local anaesthetic cream for pain-free venepuncture in laboratory animals. *Lab. Anim.* 24 (2): 142–146.

7 Chebroux, A., Leece, E.A., and Brearley, J.C. (2015). Ease of intravenous catheterization in dogs and cats: a comparative study of two peripheral catheters. *J. Small Anim. Pract.* 56 (4): 242–246.

8 Fetzer, S.J. (2002). Reducing venipuncture and intravenous insertion pain with eutectic mixture of local anesthetic: a meta-analysis. *Nurs. Res.* 51 (2): 119–124.

9 Rogers, T.L. and Ostrow, C.L. (2004). The use of EMLA cream to decrease venipuncture pain in children. *J. Pediatr. Nurs.* 19 (1): 33–39.

10 Brodeur, A., Wright, A., and Cortes, Y. (2017). Hypothermia and targeted temperature management in cats and dogs. *J. Vet. Emerg. Crit. Care* 27 (2): 151–163.

11 Clark-Price, S.C. (2015). Inadvertent perianesthetic hypothermia in small animal patients. *Vet. Clin. Small Anim.* 45 (5): 983–994.

12 Guyton, A.C. and Hall, J.E. (eds.) (2016). *Textbook of Medical Physiology*, 14e. Philadelphia: Elsevier.

13 Aarnes, T.K., Bednarski, R.M., Lerche, P. et al. (2017). Effect of pre-warming on perioperative hypothermia and anesthetic recovery in small breed dogs undergoing ovariohysterectomy. *Can. Vet. J.* 58 (2): 175–179.

14 Clark-Price, S.C., Dossin, O., Jones, K.R. et al. (2013). Comparison of three different methods to prevent heat loss in healthy dogs undergoing 90 minutes of general anesthesia. *Vet. Anaesth. Analg.* 40 (3): 280–284.

15 Machon, R.G., Raffe, M.R., and Robinson, E.P. (1999). Warming with a forced air warming blanket minimizes anesthetic-induced hypothermia in cats. *Vet. Surg.* 28 (4): 301–333.

16 Miller, R.D., Cohen, N.H., Eriksson, L.I. et al. (eds.) (2015). *Miller's Anesthesia*, 8e. St Louis, MO: Saunders Elsevier.

17 Tobias, K.M. and Johnston, S.A. (2012). *Veterinary Surgery Small Animal*. St. Louis, MO: Elsevier.

18 Fryer, K.J., Levine, J.M., Peycke, L.E. et al. (2011). Incidence of postoperative seizures with and without levetiracetam pretreatment in dogs undergoing portosystemic shunt attenuation. *J. Vet. Intern. Med.* 25 (6): 1379–1384.

19 Ahboucha, S. and Butterworth, R.F. (2004). Pathophysiology of hepatic encephalopathy: a new look at GABA from the molecular standpoint. *Metab. Brain Dis.* 19 (3–4): 331–343.

20 Goulenok, C., Bernard, B., Cadranel, J.F. et al. (2002). Flumazenil vs. placebo in hepatic encephalopathy in patients with cirrhosis: a meta-analysis. *Aliment. Pharmacol. Ther.* 16 (3): 361–372.

21 Slatter, D. (2003). *Small Animal Surgery*, 3e. Philadelphia: Saunders.

22 Fleming, J.M., Creevy, K.E., and Promislow, D.E. (2011). Mortality in North American dogs from 1984–2004: an investigation into age, size, and breed related causes of death. *J. Vet. Intern. Med.* 25: 187–198.

23 Paajanen, T.A., Oksala, N.K., Kuukasjarvi, P. et al. (2010). Short stature is associated with coronary heart disease: a systematic review of the literature and a meta-analysis. *Eur. Heart J.* 31: 1802e–1809e.

24 Diehl, K.H., Hull, R., Morton, D. et al. (2001). A good practice guide to the administration of substances and removal of blood, including routes and volumes. *J. Appl. Toxicol.* 21 (1): 15–23.

25 Thomas, J.A. and Lerche, P. (eds.) (2011). *Anesthesia and Analgesia for Veterinary Technicians*, 4e. USA: Elsevier.

26 Shin, C.W., Son, W.G., Jang, M. et al. (2018). Changes in endotracheal tube intracuff pressure and air leak pressure over time in anesthetized beagle dogs. *Vet. Anaesth. Analg.* 45 (6): 737–744.

27 Grimm, K.A., Lamont, L.A., Tranquilli, W.J. et al. (eds.) (2015). *Lumb & Jones' Veterinary Anesthesia and Analgesia*, 5e. USA: Wiley-Blackwell.

28 Briganti, A., Portela, D.A., Barsotti, G. et al. (2012). Evaluation of the endotracheal tube cuff pressure resulting from four different methods of inflation in dogs. *Vet. Anaesth. Analg.* 39 (5): 488–494.

29 Dawson, C. and Sanchez, R.F. (2016). A prospective study of the prevalence of corneal surface disease in dogs receiving prophylactic topical lubrication under general anesthesia. *Vet. Ophthalmol.* 19 (2): 124–129.

30 Park, Y.W., Son, W.G., Jeong, M.B. et al. (2013). Evaluation of risk factors for development of corneal ulcer after non-ocular surgery in dogs: 14 cases (2009–2011). *J. Am. Vet. Med. Assoc.* 242 (11): 1544–1548.

31 Gains, M.J., Grodecki, K.M., Jacobs, R.M. et al. (1995). Comparison of direct and indirect pressure measurements in anesthetized dogs. *Can. J. Vet. Res.* 59: 238–240.

32 Ypsilantis, P., Didilis, V.N., Politou, M. et al. (2005). A comparative study of invasive and oscillometric methods of arterial blood pressure measurement in the anaesthetized rabbit. *Res. Vet. Sci.* 78: 269–275.

33 Kennedy, M.J. and Barletta, M. (2015). Agreement between dopper and invasive blood pressure monitoring in anesthetized dogs weighing < 5 kg. *J. Am. Anim. Hosp. Assoc.* 51: 300–305.

34 Moll, X., Aguilar, A., Garcia, F. et al. (2018). Validity and reliability of Doppler ultrasonography and direct arterial blood pressure measurements in anaesthetized dogs weighing less than 5 kg. *Vet. Anaesth. Analg.* 45: 135–144.

35 Perrin, C., Seksel, K., and Landsberg, G.M. (2014). Appendix: drug dosage chart. *Vet. Clin. Small Anim.* 44: 629–632.

9

Brachycephalic Breeds and Anesthesia

Amber Hopkins

VCA Alameda East Veterinary Hospital, Denver, CO, USA

9.1 Introduction

Over the last decade, the number of brachycephalic pets in the UK, Australia, Brazil and North America have dramatically increased due to their increasing popularity [1, 2]. With this increase, comes the increased likelihood that a practitioner will have to anesthetize more of these patients in the years to come. With continual studies on these breeds' anatomic conformations, ability for surgical intervention, advances in monitoring and anesthetic drugs; the risks associated with anesthetizing these breeds can certainly be dramatically reduced. There is a moderately long list of canine brachycephalic breeds depending on the measuring metric used (Table 9.1), but breeds of particular concern are the French Bulldog, English Bulldog, and Pug. There are a few brachycephalic feline breeds, with the Persian and Himalayan being most common.

The term brachycephalic means short skull. There are different metrics published describing what defines a brachycephalic breed but no established gold standard. One of these metrics is called the cephalic index, which is the ratio between the width and length of the skull. Regardless, brachycephalic breeds have a skull that is shortened in the rostro-caudal direction with a wider interzygomatic width. Skeletal growth is reported to be reduced secondary to genetic, hormonal deficits or epiphyseal dysfunction of bones [3]. While this premature ankylosis of the basicranial epiphyseal cartilage results in a shortened longitudinal axis of the bones of skull, the associated soft tissues develop normally, causing excess tissue in a small cavity of bone structure, leading to crowding and obstruction of the upper airway [4].

This chapter will discuss brachycephalic airway syndrome (BAS), its consequences, peri-anesthetic period (pre, intra and post) evaluation of the patient, peri-anesthetic considerations and how to minimize their peri-anesthetic risks.

9.2 Brachycephalic Airway Syndrome (BAS) Pathophysiology

BAS is also known as brachycephalic syndrome (BS) and brachycephalic obstructive airway syndrome (BOAS). Primary airway abnormalities that are commonly associated with this syndrome include elongated soft palate, stenotic nares and aberrant nasopharyngeal turbinates (Figures 9.1 and 9.2). Though not technically considered to be part of the BAS, many of these patients also

Breed Predispositions to Dental and Oral Disease in Dogs, First Edition. Edited by Brook A. Niemiec.
© 2021 John Wiley & Sons, Inc. Published 2021 by John Wiley & Sons, Inc.

Table 9.1 Commonly reported brachycephalic breeds.

Canine	Feline
French Bulldog	Persian
English Bulldog	Himalayan
Pug	Burmese
Boston Terrier	Exotic short hair
Brussels Griffon	
Affenpinscher	
Japanese Chin	
King Charles Cavalier	
Shih Tzu	
Mastiff	
Dogue de Bordeaux	

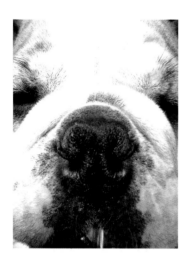

Figure 9.1 Pre-surgical stenotic nares. Source: Image William Snell.

have hypoplastic trachea, with English Bulldogs being overrepresented [5–9]. Secondary sequelae include Stage I laryngeal collapse (everted laryngeal saccules) which may progress to Stage III laryngeal collapse and lower airway dysfunction [10]. Common clinical signs in these patients include dyspnea, exercise intolerance, gastrointestinal (GI) signs, stridor, snoring, syncope, heat exhaustion and cyanosis [11].

All of the upper respiratory tract abnormalities result in narrowing of the airway passages, restriction of airflow and increased resistance to flow. According to Poiseuille's Law, if there is a 50% reduction in the diameter of a tube, there is a 16-fold increase in resistance and therefore increased intraluminal pressure. This increased pressure leads to swelling and edema of upper airway structures, further narrowing of the airways, causing decreased ability to dissipate heat and worsening of the airway obstruction [1, 11]. These changes in their upper airway can, over time, result in lower airway disease, most commonly aspiration pneumonia and/or post-obstructive pulmonary edema [5, 12–14]. Additionally, these breeds also often suffer from a multitude of other anatomic

Figure 9.2 Elongated soft palate; palate extending past the epiglottis. Source: Image courtesy of Amber Hopkins.

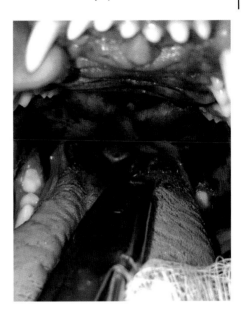

abnormalities, that when combined, complicate the peri-anesthetic period for these patients and potentially increase their anesthetic risks.

9.3   Other Pre-existing Conditions in the Brachycephalic Patient

The respiratory apparatus is the most commonly affected system and generally the one that has the most significant impact on the patient's life. However, many other body systems in these breeds can also be affected which may further complicate anesthesia.

9.3.1   Gastrointestinal

The prevalence rate of GI disease in patients with BOAS has been shown to be as high as 97.3% and largely correlates with severity of respiratory disease [15]. Underlying GI diseases which were identified included: distal esophagitis, gastroesophageal reflux and duodenitis based on endoscopic and histopathologic examination [15]. Later, Poncet et al. determined that brachycephalic patients that had correction of their upper airway abnormalities and medical management of their GI disease, had over 94% improvement in their GI clinical signs [16]. This demonstrates that GI disease may in fact be secondary to the upper respiratory disease.

Congenital hiatal hernias have been reported in the English and French Bulldogs and may also be a sequela to BOAS, though supporting evidence for that is scant. It is theorized that due to increased abdominal inspiratory effort, the pressure gradient between the thorax and the abdomen is also increased, causing cranial displacement of the esophageal hiatus, gastroesophageal reflux, and esophagitis [11, 17].

These disease processes can increase the patient risk for regurgitation and aspiration pneumonia, which can be life-threatening. Understanding the significant correlation and consequences of these two disease processes, gives insight as to more recent recommendations for medical management of their GI disease prior to anesthesia and/or surgery. This will be discussed in detail later in the chapter.

9.3.2 Body Conformation and Condition Score

In human patients, obesity plays a large role in increasing the risk of regurgitation and worsening of airway obstruction in patients with obstructive sleep apnea. In dogs the literature is varied, and while Lamata et al. did find a correlation between body weight and risk for regurgitation [18], there have been no supporting studies that obesity worsens BOAS. Their barrel-chested conformation, higher propensity for obesity and the potential for them to be in dorsal recumbency during surgery, however, can decrease their ability to adequately ventilate spontaneously during anesthesia. Brachycephalics have also been described as having a lower tidal volume, which limits alveolar gas exchange and increases the risk for respiratory acidosis [19]. Mechanical ventilation should be considered, when available, to maximize carbon dioxide elimination and proper oxygen exchange.

9.3.3 Cardiovascular

In humans, obstructive airway syndromes have been associated with a higher incidence of cardiac disease and therefore higher morbidity and mortality. However, though extensive study on this has not been performed in the brachycephalic canine breeds, one study did not show evidence of increased risk in dogs with BSOA [20]. With that said, Boxers have been documented to have a higher incidence of arrhythmogenic right ventricular cardiomyopathy (ARVC) and ventricular tachycardia, which has also been documented in English Bulldogs [21]. Additionally, pulmonic stenosis, which is the third most common congenital defect in dogs, includes English Bulldogs as an overrepresented breed [22]. Therefore, a thorough physical exam and history prior to anesthesia are crucial, while a pre-anesthetic ECG and echocardiogram may also be of benefit.

9.3.4 Ocular

Ocular conformation in these breeds predisposes them to potential injury, corneal ulceration and potentially globe prolapse. Care should be taken in handling and restraint, and proactive measures to maintain protection and lubrication of their corneas during anesthetic and surgical procedures instituted. It has also been established that decreased tear production is a risk factor for corneal ulceration or erosion and that general anesthesia significantly decreases tear production. Further, lengthy procedures, lateral positioning, and procedures of the head all increase the risk of corneal damage [23]. Based on the variable residence time of ocular lubricants, dependent on their formulation and concentration, as well as the likelihood of chemical, debris and physical contact of the cornea during dental procedures, it is recommended that eyes be lubricated every 30 minutes. It is also worth noting that, tear production remains decreased for up to 24 hours post-anesthesia and thus prescription of eye lubrication during that time may be of benefit, particularly to high risk patients [24].

9.4 Pre-anesthetic Considerations

There are several factors that affect how a higher risk patient will do during the peri-anesthetic period, including: patient history and assessment, diagnostic results, planned procedure, drug selection, anesthetic monitoring, maintenance, and recovery. Below is a discussion of anesthetic planning and management.

9.4.1 Patient History, Physical Examination, and Recommended Diagnostics

A complete patient history is of utmost importance. Determining the severity of upper and lower respiratory compromise is vital. Particular questions of importance include any changes in respiratory sound or effort, if so, does it worsen with exercise? Does the patient have evidence of exercise intolerance or intolerance to heat? Is there a history of coughing, vomiting or regurgitation and has the patient ever demonstrated cyanosis or collapse? These answers will give some insight as to how significantly the patient is affected by its BOAS, if there is reason to be concerned that the patient has underlying gastrointestinal disease, what pre-anesthetic diagnostics should be considered, and what pre-anesthetic management should be implemented. Patients with underlying gastrointestinal disease are at a higher risk for esophagitis, regurgitation and therefore aspiration pneumonia. If medical management is implemented prior to anesthesia, post-operative prognosis is improved [15, 16].

It is also important to inquire as to whether the patient has any other co-morbidities, such as renal hepatic or cardiovascular disease, or any endocrinopathies. It is all too often that we focus on the obvious abnormality without considering the whole picture. With that, it is vital to know what medications the patient is currently taking and how those may interfere with or be interfered with by the anesthetic drugs. Lastly, always inquire about the past anesthetic or surgical procedures. Knowing if the patient had anesthetic complications, how they were managed, if management corrected the anesthetic issue, did the patient recover well or have a longer than expected recovery, all can aid in making the best anesthetic plan and minimize the risk of similar complications occurring again. Previous surgeries can also affect the plan and management for your patient. For example, if your patient had a previous lung lobectomy, you would not use the same tidal volume for mechanical ventilation as a patient that had not had a lung resection.

Physical examination will give you a tremendous amount of information. A patient that demonstrates stertor, a lower pitched noise, is usually associated with issues of the nasopharynx and pharynx. Stridor, which is a higher pitched noise, can be a strong indicator of laryngeal collapse [25]. If the patient has not already had a full oral/laryngeal exam, it should be done during the induction phase of anesthesia. Visual assessment of the nares and listening for any whistling may alert the practitioner of the risk of stenotic nares and potential for obstruction of nasal airflow. Auscultation of the thorax may also alert you to any potential concerns for lower airway disease, murmurs, or arrhythmias.

Typically, prior to any general anesthesia, some form of bloodwork should be performed to rule out evidence of anemia, hepatic, renal and other systemic diseases. Red blood cells are responsible for transport of oxygen to the tissues, the liver metabolizes most drugs, and the kidneys are responsible for elimination of both the primary drug and metabolites for many of the commonly used anesthetic drugs. Dysfunction of these organs can lead to more profound drug effects and longer recovery times. Additionally, these patients often have higher oxygen demands and therefore rely more heavily on red blood cell delivery of oxygen to vital organs.

Thoracic radiographs are often recommended in the brachycephalic patient due to their higher risk for aspiration pneumonia and risk for gastrointestinal abnormalities such as hiatal hernia. Pre-operative ECG can also be considered particularly in breeds at a higher predisposition for arrhythmogenic diseases, e.g. Boxers with a higher incidence of ARVC. Evaluation of tracheal diameter, particularly in English Bulldogs, can help determine what size endotracheal tube may be most appropriate and minimize delays in intubation, as these breeds are predisposed to significantly smaller tracheas compared to other breeds of similar body size.

9.4.2 Procedural Considerations

This chapter's focus is on patients presenting for dental procedures. This could include anything from a professional dental cleaning to major maxillofacial surgery. Analgesia should always be a part of the anesthetic plan. It is of particular importance in these patients, to have some idea of the degree of anticipated pain to determine the most appropriate analgesic and also minimize the use of drugs that may induce vomiting and nausea. If extractions or more invasive excision of tissue is suspected, the addition of local blocks can be very beneficial.

9.4.3 Drug Considerations

Pre-anesthetic drug choices include both those indicated for medical management of underlying diseases, as well as those specific for sedation, minimum alveolar concentration (MAC) reduction and pain relief.

9.4.3.1 Gastrointestinal Drugs

Gastroprotectants and prokinetics are recommended for pre-anesthetic medical management for these patients (Table 9.2). These recommendations address both these patients' high prevalence of upper and lower gastrointestinal disease, as well as relaxation of the lower esophageal sphincter associated with many injectable anesthetic drugs [28]. The 2018 ACVIM consensus statement determined that proton pump inhibitors (PPIs) are superior to H_2RA in increasing gastric pH [29]. Ideally, these patients are prescribed a PPI to start a day or two prior to presenting for anesthesia. If this is not possible, an injectable PPI, such as esomeprazole or pantoprazole IV is preferred but famotidine, an inexpensive injectable H_2RA, may be a reasonable choice for immediate and short-term use [29]. Prokinetics are also recommended to reduce the incidence of gastroesophageal reflux. Cisapride has been demonstrated to be superior to metoclopramide in increasing gastric emptying and increasing lower esophageal sphincter tone [26]. Post-operative nausea and vomiting has been well-documented and is thought to be associated with volatile anesthetics, opioids, body weight and type of procedure [18, 28]. Anti-emetics have therefore been suggested as part of the pre-anesthetic plan in these patients. Maropitant, a selective neurokinin-1 (NK-1) antagonist, blocks the binding of the neurotransmitter Substance P, which is found in high concentrations in the chemoreceptor trigger zone and the vomiting center and considered a key component in vomiting. Several studies have demonstrated a reduction in nausea and vomiting secondary to opioids, as well as a faster return to eating post-operatively when maropitant was used pre-operatively [30]. Ideally, all of these medications are started a few days prior and continued a few days post-surgery, however if the client is unable to start these medications before the day of surgery, they or drugs in their same drug class can be administered the day of and still have significant benefit.

9.4.3.2 Pre-anesthetics

As was discussed earlier, brachycephalic breeds have higher than normal vasovagal tone [31]. Historically, pre-anesthetic use of anticholinergics was recommended in these breeds, to minimize the effects of parasympathomimetic drugs and risk of vagal events. Today, preemptive use of anticholinergics is no longer routinely recommended due to the risk of tachyarrhythmias, increased myocardial workload and oxygen demand, decreases in gastrointestinal motility and decreased esophageal sphincter tone [28, 32]. It is recommended, however, to monitor these patients closely after premedication, as well as during induction and recovery, and to have a dose of atropine calculated and easily accessible in the event a vagal event occurs. In addition, some clinicians will premedicate

Table 9.2 Gastroprotectant and prokinetic doses.

Drug	MOA	Canine dose	CRI rate
Omeprazole	PPI	$1\,\text{mg}\,\text{kg}^{-1}$ PO	
Esomeprazole	PPI	$1\,\text{mg}\,\text{kg}^{-1}$ IV, PO	
Pantoprazole	PPI	$1\,\text{mg}\,\text{kg}^{-1}$ IV	
Famotidine	H2RA	$0.5–1\,\text{mg}\,\text{kg}^{-1}$ IV	
Cisapride	Prokinetic	$0.1–1.0\,\text{mg}\,\text{kg}^{-1}$ PO/IV	
Metaclopramide	Prokinetic	$1\,\text{mg}\,\text{kg}^{-1}$ IV	$1\,\text{mg}\,(\text{kg}\,\text{h})^{-1}$

IV administration should ideally occur 2–4 h prior to administration of pre-anesthetic drugs such as sedatives or analgesics [26, 27].
MOA: mechanism of action; CRI: constant rate infusion.
Source: Table compiled using multiple sources: Zacuto, AC., Marks, SL., Osborn, J. et al. (2012) The influence of esomeprazole and cisapride on gastroesophageal reflux during anesthesia in dogs. J Vet Intern Med 26(3): 518–525; Ogden, J., Ovbey, D., Saile, K. (2019) Effects of preoperative cisapride on postoperative aspiration pneumonia in dogs with laryngeal paralysis. J Small Anim Pract 60(3): 183–190.

patients with alpha 2 agonists which have been demonstrated to cause a reflex bradycardia secondary to increases in systemic blood pressure. Congdon et al. demonstrated that the concurrent use of dexmedetomidine and atropine resulted in increased oxygen consumption, hypertension and increased cardiac arrhythmias compared to those patients that received only dexmedetomidine [33]. The pre-anesthetic administration of steroids, particularly dexamethasone ($0.05–2\,\text{mg}\,\text{kg}^{-1}$) has also been recommended by some [14, 34] though there is limited evidence to support its usefulness in preventing post-anesthetic airway obstruction.

Ideally, management of pain begins before the pain stimulus occurs. When this does not occur, analgesic measures should be implemented as soon as possible. Today we have many options for peri-operative pain management. NSAIDs, opioids, local anesthetics and alpha 2 agonists are the most commonly used peri-operative analgesics. Controversy surrounds the use of NSAIDs in these patients, due to the high incidence of underlying gastrointestinal disease as well as the potential need for post-operative steroids if laryngeal or pharyngeal edema results in airway obstruction. In this author's opinion, should steroids not be used perioperatively and the patient has no documented gastrointestinal or renal disease, NSAID should still be considered postoperatively.

Pure mu opioids are excellent analgesics but also have a variety of negative side effects such as excessive sedation, dysphoria, panting, respiratory depression, decreased GI motility, nausea, and vomiting [32]. Opioids that predispose patients to vomiting (e.g. morphine, hydromorphone) should be used with caution, always used with preemptive anti-emetics and the patient closely monitored for evidence of nausea and vomiting. Methadone is widely preferred, due to its reliable analgesia and minimal incidence of nausea, vomiting or panting, but is very costly and at the time of writing this chapter, was difficult to acquire for many hospitals. Partial agonists, such as buprenorphine, have fewer side effects and provide similar analgesia to morphine, however, with a lower maximal effect. It is highly competitive for the mu receptor resulting in significantly higher doses of naloxone for reversal, if needed. Knowing the anticipated degree of pain will help choose the most appropriate opioid. If a significant amount of pain is expected, a pure mu over a partial agonist may be recommended.

Pre-emptive analgesia prevents both the central sensitization of the pain pathways and the release of peripheral chemicals that disrupt tissue healing [35]. Regional anesthesia of the oral cavity should be used prior to disruption of the tissues whenever possible, as they provide multimodal pain control, MAC reduction, minimize the need for high doses of opioids and avoid sedation, nausea and vomiting secondary to other systemic analgesics. Bupivacaine, ropivacaine and lidocaine are the most common local anesthetics used for this purpose. Lidocaine has the advantage of a rapid on set of action but also has a shorter duration of action. Bupivacaine and ropivacaine both have a prolonged onset but a far longer duration of action. Epinephrine, a vasoconstrictor, is often combined with the local anesthetic to help reduce hemorrhage, prolong the duration and reduce systemic uptake of the local anesthetic. Systemic uptake can occur, resulting in hypertension and tachycardia so these parameters should be watched closely after administration.

Sedation and anxiolysis is of utmost importance in the brachycephalic patient to minimize stress, ease catheter placement and minimize risk of airway obstruction. When using any sedation, is important to monitor them closely after premedication, as many of these drugs can cause naso and pharyngeal muscle relaxation, excessive sedation and risk of compromise of the upper airway. Phenothiazines such as acepromazine are commonly used at low doses (0.01 mg kg^{-1}), to provide mild tranquilization.

Benzodiazepines have minimal effects on cardiovascular function, are reversible, and can be safely used for premedication or as a co-induction agent in many patients. It is important to note, however, that many patients can have paradoxical excitatory reactions to benzodiazepines. In addition, they can promote muscle relaxation which could predispose them to airway compromise. They have also been demonstrated to decrease lower esophageal sphincter tone, which increases the risk of regurgitation under anesthesia. Finally, in human patients with obstructive sleep apnea, this class of drugs increases their risk for adverse respiratory events and respiratory failure [28, 36]. If benzodiazepines are used, flumazenil should be available for benzodiazepine reversal if needed in recovery.

Alpha 2 agonists at very low (1–2 µg kg^{-1}) doses can provide reliable sedation and some additional analgesia. They can also cause a reflex bradycardia and hypoventilation. As these patients are prone to higher vagal tone and slower heart rates to begin with and alpha 2 agonists can cause excess sedation, patients should be very closely monitored after administration. Alpha 2 agonists are reversible, and thus reversal agents should be available and easily accessible.

9.4.3.3 Induction

Studies comparing propofol and alfaxalone have demonstrated very similar pharmacodynamics and similar usefulness for laryngeal exams in dogs, when premedicated with acepromazine and butorphanol [37]. Interestingly however, when evaluating risk factors for regurgitation in anesthetized dogs, propofol has a significantly higher incidence of regurgitation compared to those induced with alfaxalone [18]. This may suggest that alfaxalone should be considered in patients at a higher risk for regurgitation. Propofol has been found to decrease lower esophageal sphincter tone, which would increase risk for regurgitation [38].

9.5 Anesthetic Management

There is some debate as to whether these patients should have a longer or shorter food and water fasting time. Historically it was recommended that BAS patients be fasted longer (up to 24 hours) due to their higher risk for vomiting, regurgitation and aspiration. However, more recent studies indicate that feeding a small amount of canned food three hours before anesthesia did not increase gastric content volume and actually reduced the incidence of gastroesophageal reflux [39, 40]. It is worth noting that these studies were not performed in brachycephalic patients nor in patients with a history of gastroesophageal disease, which may complicate the decision to feed high-risk patients closer to the time of induction.

While all dogs and cats benefit from the reduction of pre-anesthetic stress, it is vital to minimize anxiety and practice gentle and stress-free handling in this population of patients (see Chapter 6). Premedication with sedatives and analgesics can be very beneficial and allow for less restraint, particularly of their cervical region, and easier placement of intravenous catheters.

Once sedated, these patients should be monitored closely for any signs of vomiting, regurgitation or respiratory distress. Intravenous catheterization can also be difficult in these breeds, due not only to the conformation of their limbs but due to their propensity for very thick skin.

Preoxygenation for three to five minutes should be attempted in every patient, to increase arterial oxygen content and saturation and prolong the time before desaturation occurs. This is best accomplished with a snug fitting mask and $3–5\,l\,min^{-1}$ oxygen [41]. Brachycephalic breeds have a lower than normal oxygen concentration compared to non-brachycephalic breeds awake and at rest, meaning they are predisposed to more rapid desaturation when compared to a non-brachycephalic breed [19]. Additionally, since some of these patients may already have a hypoplastic trachea and/or swelling of the airway tissues, intubation may be more difficult and take longer to accomplish, so maximizing their residual oxygen capacity is even more important. If, however, this technique causes more stress and struggling for the patient, modifications of the technique or discontinuing it may outweigh its benefits.

Pre-induction preparation should ideally include the use of a patient safety checklist to assure all diagnostics have been performed and reviewed by the clinician, the anesthetic machine and monitoring equipment have been checked, and all necessary anesthesia and surgical equipment are ready. Studies done by the World Health Organization have demonstrated a significant decrease in morbidity and mortality, secondary to human associated medical mistakes, when patient safety checklists are used prior to anesthesia [42]. This trend is becoming more common in the veterinary industry. As intubation can be more difficult, a long laryngoscope blade with a bright light, multiple sized and pre-checked endotracheal tubes, a stylet, a tongue depressor, gauze and a syringe for inflation of the endotracheal tube cuff should already be at hand. A full examination of the airway on induction should be completed to determine if any proximal airway abnormalities are present. If any abnormalities are noted, they may be of a concern on recovery and surgical intervention should be discussed with the client when necessary. Sternal recumbency is indicated for induction for many reasons, including: ability for complete evaluation of the oral cavity, intubation is often easier and more rapid, and the risk of aspiration if patient regurgitates is reduced compared to induction in lateral recumbency. Immediately upon intubation and before the volatile anesthetic is turned on, the endotracheal tube cuff should be checked for a leak and inflated only enough to occlude airflow around the tube. It is important to assure a secure occlusion to prevent the aspiration of any regurgitant material or water/debris associated with the dental procedure. It is also important to not over inflate the endotracheal tube cuff, as this can predispose patients to tracheal irritation, inflammation, coughing, tracheal tears and strictures which can worsen their airway issues and potentially lead to death [43].

Maintenance of general anesthesia can be accomplished with the use of volatile anesthetics, PIVA (partial intravenous anesthesia) or TIVA (total intravenous anesthesia), depending on any other co-morbidities and patient needs. There is no perfect drug protocol but rather preferred and less preferred drugs, based on each individual's history, other co-morbidities and procedure.

As mentioned earlier, these patients may be more prone to intra-operative panting and hypoventilation and may therefore require mechanical ventilation. Blood pressure monitoring can also be a challenge in these patients. Many of these breeds have no tail and the conformation of both their front and hind limbs make finding an appropriate fitting blood pressure cuff more challenging. There have been no specific studies done in brachycephalic breeds, to determine the most accurate placement of blood pressure cuff, however, non-invasive blood pressure readings taken below the hock, over the dorsal pedal artery, can be the easiest to obtain and the tail used if available. Monitoring invasive blood pressures via an arterial catheter is ideal, when possible can be very adventitious. Other important monitoring includes pulse oximetry, end-tidal carbon dioxide, electrocardiography and core body temperature.

9.6 Anesthetic Recovery

It is not uncommon to have a reasonable level of fear during the anesthetic period, as the patient's life is literally in your hands. However, there is sometimes a misconception that once the procedure is done and the patient is awake that your job is done, and you can breathe a sigh of relief that the patient made it through. While that does indicate a job well done, it is also not the period on the end of the sentence. In all patients, but especially brachycephalic breeds, the recovery period is arguably the most important a part of the peri-anesthetic time. In fact, peri-anesthetic deaths have been reported to be the highest in the recovery period and often within the first three hours after extubation [44]. This is likely multifactorial:

1. Once the patient is extubated, there is no longer an assured and protected airway.
2. These patients are, in many cases, hypothermic which may slow recovery and excretion of anesthetic drugs.
3. They no longer have monitoring equipment attached to them and once extubated are often left alone without much visual or hands-on monitoring.
4. When a patient wakes up poorly, it is commonplace to give them more drugs and then walk away from them, leaving them at risk for unintended excess sedation, resulting in airway obstruction, hypoventilation, hypoxemia, regurgitation and aspiration.

All patients should have active monitoring and vitals taken every 15-30 minutes for the first three hours after extubation, to ensure that they are warming and recovering appropriately. If the patient has just received additional sedation medication, is very cold or is a high-risk patient, they should be evaluated more frequently. For BAS patients specifically, the recovery process should be more involved. It is recommended that these patients be recovered in sternal recumbency, on a table or in a cage with a technician dedicated to them. At the very minimum, the patient should have pulse oximetry attached and ideally supplemental oxygen provided until extubated and potentially even after extubation (whenever possible). The patient should remain in sternal recumbency after recovery when possible. Extubation should not occur until the patient is actively swallowing and will no longer tolerate intubation.

Immediately after extubation, these patients should be watched closely by a dedicated technician for any evidence of increased vagal tone, cyanosis, regurgitation, hypoventilation, airway obstruction or excessive sedation for a period of at least 15–30 minutes. The anesthetist should always have extra induction drugs, a laryngoscope and extra endotracheal tubes in the event the patient obstructs its airway and needs re-intubation. If the patient recovers as dysphoric or agitated, reversal of any benzodiazepines is a good first step. Mild sedation with acepromazine or micro-doses of dexmedetomidine may also be indicated, however, the patient should be monitored for over-sedation and secondary signs of airway obstruction hypoventilation or lack of ability to swallow. If the patient is suspected to have swelling/edema of the upper airway, anti-inflammatory doses of steroids may be beneficial, if not otherwise contraindicated. There should always be a discussion with the client prior to anesthesia that in more advanced airway disease, surgical correction of the airway may be necessary if recovery does not go well and while rare, there is always a chance that tracheostomy and/or mechanical ventilation will be indicated if extubation cannot be safely achieved.

9.7 Conclusion

Brachycephalic breeds can be anesthetized safely, however, they do have many inherent anesthetic risk factors. Pre-anesthesia workup, a thorough history and physical exam, thorough preparation, proper anesthetic protocols, continuous and detailed monitoring (including the post-operative period) and the use of gastroprotectants can all help minimize the risk to the patient. Further, the simple fact of being a brachycephalic breed should not preclude the patient from receiving proper dental care. A risk: benefit ratio should be carried out on each patient. Though anesthesia in the patients are often uneventful, a discussion with the owner prior to the procedure to explain the potential risks for recovery should also be done ahead of time and a post-anesthetic plan discussed in the event the recovery process becomes complicated. Finally, referral for therapy to a facility where an anesthesiologist and/or ECC/ICU should be offered any time the practitioner is uncomfortable with proceeding with anesthesia.

References

1 Fawcett, A., Barrs, V., Awad, M. et al. (2019). Consequences and management of canine brachycephaly in veterinary practice: perspectives from Australian veterinarians and veterinary specialists. *Animals* 9 (1). 2.

2 Lodato, D. and Hedlund, C.S. (2012). Brachycephalic airway syndrome: management. *Compend. Contin. Educ. Vet.* 34 (8): E1–E8.

3 Schmidt, M.J., Amort, K.H., Failing, K. et al. (2014). Comparison of the endocranial- and brain volumes in brachycephalic dogs, mesaticephalic dogs and cavalier king Charles spaniels in relation to their body weight. *Acta Vet. Scand.* 56 (1): 30.

4 Stockard, C.R. *The Genetic and Endocrinic Basis for Differences in form and Behavior: As Elucidated by Studies of Contrasted Pure-line Dog Breeds and Their Hybrids*, vol. 19. 1: The Wistar Institute of Anatomy and Biology.

5 Wykes, P.M. (1991). Brachycephalic airway obstructive syndrome. *Probl. Vet. Med.* 3 (2): 188–197.

6 Rozanski, E. and Chan, D.L. (2005). Approach to the patient with respiratory distress. *Vet. Clin. North Am. Small Anim. Pract.* 35 (2): 307–317.

7 Dupre, G. (2008). Brachycephalic syndrome: new knowledge, new treatments. *Proceedings of the 33rd World Small Anim Vet Assoc & 14th FECAVA,* Dublin, Ireland. (20–24 August 2008). WSAVA.

8 Pink, J.J., Doyle, R.S., Hughes, J.M. et al. (2006). Laryngeal collapse in seven brachycephalic puppies. *J. Small Anim. Pract.* 47 (3): 131–135.

9 Ginn, J.A., Kumar, M.S., McKiernan, B.C. et al. (2008). Nasopharyngeal turbinates in brachycephalic dogs and cats. *J. Am. Anim. Hosp. Assoc.* 44 (5): 243–249.

10 Emmerson, T. (2014). Brachycephalic obstructive airway syndrome: a growing problem. *J. Small Anim. Pract.* 55 (11): 543–544.

11 Packer, R. and Tivers, M. (2015). Strategies for the management and prevention of conformation-related respiratory disorders in brachycephalic dogs. *Vet. Med. Res. Rep.* 6: 219–232.

12 Darcy, H.P., Humm, K., and Haar, G. (2018). Retrospective analysis of incidence, clinical features, potential risk factors, and prognostic indicators for aspiration pneumonia in three brachycephalic dog breeds. *J. Am. Vet. Med. Assoc.* 253 (7): 869–876.

13 Seim, H.B. (2001). Brachycephalic syndrome. *Proceedings of the 13th Atlantic Coast Veterinary Conference,* Atlantic City, NJ (9–11 October 2001). ACVC.

14 Hendricks, J.C. (1992). Brachycephalic airway syndrome. *Vet. Clin. North Am. Small Anim. Pract.* 22 (5): 1145–1153.

15 Poncet, C.M., Dupre, G.P., Freiche, V.G. et al. (2005). Prevalence of gastrointestinal tract lesions in 73 brachycephalic dogs with upper respiratory syndrome. *J. Small Anim. Pract.* 46 (6): 273–279.

16 Poncet, C.M., Dupre, G.P., Freiche, V.G. et al. (2006). Long-term results of upper respiratory syndrome surgery and gastrointestinal tract medical treatment in 51 brachycephalic dogs. *J. Small Anim. Pract.* 47 (3): 137–142.

17 Reeve, E.J., Sutton, D., Friend, E.J. et al. (2017). Documenting the prevalence of hiatal hernia and oesophageal abnormalities in brachycephalic dogs using fluoroscopy. *J. Small Anim. Pract.* 58 (12): 703–708.

18 Lamata, C., Loughton, V., Jones, M. et al. (2012). The risk of passive regurgitation during general anaesthesia in a population of referred dogs in the UK. *Vet. Anaesth. Analg.* 39 (3): 266–274.

19 Hoareau, G.L., Mellema, M., and Silverstein, D.C. (2011). Indication, management and outcome of brachycephalic dogs requiring mechanical ventilation. *J. Vet. Emerg. Crit. Care* 21 (3): 226–235.

20 Planellas, M., Cuenca, R., Tabar, M.D. et al. (2012). Evaluation of C-reactive protein, Haptoglobin and cardiac troponin 1 levels in brachycephalic dogs with upper airway obstructive syndrome. *BMC Vet. Res.* 8: 152.

21 Santilli, R.A., Bontempi, L.V., and Perego, M. (2011). Ventricular tachycardia in English bulldogs with localized right ventricular outflow tract enlargement. *J. Small Anim. Pract.* 52 (11): 574–580.

22 Ramos, R.V., Monterio-Steagall, B.P., and Steagall, P.V.M. (2012). Management and complications of anaesthesia during balloon valvuloplasty for pulmonic stenosis in dogs: 39 cases (2000–2012). *J. Small Anim. Pract.* 55 (4): 207–212.

23 Dawson, C. and Sanchez, R.F. (2016). A prospective study of the prevalence of corneal surface disease in dogs receiving prophylactic topical lubrication under general anesthesia. *Vet. Ophthalmol.* 19 (2): 124–129.

24 Park, Y.W., Son, W.G., Jeong, M.B. et al. (2013). Evaluation of risk factors for development of corneal ulcer after non-ocular surgery in dogs: 14 cases (2009-2011). *J. Am. Vet. Med. Assoc.* 242 (11): 1544–1548.

25 Riggs, J., Liu, N.C., Sutton, D.R. et al. (2019). Validation of exercise testing and laryngeal auscultation for grading brachycephalic obstructive airway syndrome in pugs, French bulldogs, and English bulldogs by using whole-body barometric plethysmography. *Vet. Surg.*: 1–9. https://doi .org/10.1111/vsu.13159.

26 Zacuto, A.C., Marks, S.L., Osborn, J. et al. (2012). The influence of esomeprazole and cisapride on gastroesophageal reflux during anesthesia in dogs. *J. Vet. Intern. Med.* 26 (3): 518–525.

27 Ogden, J., Ovbey, D., and Saile, K. (2019). Effects of preoperative cisapride on postoperative aspiration pneumonia in dogs with laryngeal paralysis. *J. Small Anim. Pract.* 60 (3): 183–190.

28 Rodríguez-Alarcón, C.A., Beristain-Ruiz, D.M., Rivera-Barreno, R. et al. (2015). Gastroesophageal reflux in anesthetized dogs: a review. *Rev. Colomb. Cienc. Pecu.* 28: 144–155.

29 Marks, S.L., Kook, P.H., Papich, M.G. et al. (2018). ACVIM consensus statement: support for rational administration of gastrointestinal protectants to dogs and cats. *J. Vet. Intern. Med.*: 1–18. https://doi.org/10.1111/jvim.15337.

30 Hay Kraus, B.L. (2017). Spotlight on the perioperative use of maropitant citrate. *Vet. Med. Res. Rep.* 8: 41–51. https://doi.org/10.2147/VMRR.S126469.

31 Doxey, S. and Boswood, A. (2004). Differences between breeds of dog in a measure of heart rate variability. *Vet. Rec.* 154 (23): 713–717.

32 Grimm, K.A., Lamont, L.A., Tranquilli, W.J. et al. (2015). *Veterinary Anesthesia and Analgesia*, 5e Lumb and Jones. Oxford: Wiley.

33 Congdon, J.M., Marquez, M., Niyom, S. et al. (2011). Evaluation of the sedative and cardiovascular effects of intramuscular administration of dexmedetomidine with and without concurrent atropine administration in dogs. *J. Am. Vet. Med. Assoc.* 239 (1): 81–89.

34 Fossum, T.W., Hedlund, C.S., Hulse, D.A. et al. (2002). Surgery of the upper airway system. In: *Small Animal Surgery*, 2e, 716–759. St. Louis, MO: Mosby.

35 Gaynor, J.S. and Muir, W.W. (2009). *Handbook of Veterinary Pain Management*, 2e. St. Louis, Missouri: Mosby.

36 Wang, S.H., Chen, W.S., Tang, S.E. et al. (2019). Benzodiazepines associated with acute respiratory failure in patients with obstructive sleep Apnea. *Front. Pharmacol.* 9: 1513. https://doi.org/10.3389/fphar.2018.01513.

37 Radkey, D.I., Hardie, R.J., and Smith, L.J. (2018). Comparison of the effects of alfaxalone and propofol with acepromazine, butorphanol and/or doxapram on laryngeal motion and quality of examination in dogs. *Vet. Anaesth. Analg.* 45 (3): 241–249.

38 Raptopoulos, D. and Galatos, A.D. (1997). Gastro-oesophageal reflux during anaesthesia induced with either thiopentone or propofol in the dog. *Vet. Anaesth. Analg.* 24: 20–22.

39 Savvas, I., Raptopoulos, D., and Rallis, T. (2016). A "light meal" three hours preoperatively decreases the incidence of gastro-esophageal reflux in dogs. *J. Am. Anim. Hosp. Assoc.* 52 (6): 357–363.

40 Savvas, I., Rallis, T., and Raptopoulos, D. (2009). The effect of pre-anaesthetic fasting time and type of food on gastric content volume and acidity in dogs. *Vet. Anaesth. Analg.* 36 (6): 539–546.

41 McNally, E.M., Robertson, S.A., and Pablo, L.S. (2009). Comparison of time to desaturation between preoxygenated and nonpreoxygenated dogs following sedation with acepromazine maleate and morphine and induction of anesthesia with propofol. *Am. J. Vet. Res.* 70 (11): 1333–1338.

42 Haynes, A.B., Weiser, T.G., Berry, W.R. et al. (2009). A surgical safety checklist to reduce morbidity and mortality in a global population. *N. Engl. J. Med.* 360 (5): 491–499.

43 Briganti, A., Porteia, D.A., Barsotti, G. et al. (2012). Evaluation of the endotracheal tube cuff pressure resulting from four different methods of inflation in dogs. *Vet. Anaesth. Analg.* 39 (5): 488–494.

44 Brodbelt, D., Blissitt, K., Hammond, R. et al. (2008). The risk of death: the confidential enquiry into perioperative small animal fatalities. *Vet. Anaesth. Analg.* 35 (5): 365–373.

10

Periodontal Therapy in Small and Toy Breed Dogs

Brook A. Niemiec

Veterinary Dental Specialties and Oral Surgery, San Diego, CA, USA

Proper treatment of periodontal disease is the same in all dogs (and species for that matter): plaque control [1, 2]. While there is a strong genetic predisposition, plaque is what initiates periodontal disease [3–5]. Without plaque, there is no infection to start the inflammatory cascade. Plaque control is achieved by a combination of routine professional dental cleanings, homecare, periodontal surgery, and extraction (depending on the level of disease) [6].

The major difference between at risk (small breed dogs as well as greyhounds and Cavalier King Charles Spaniels [CKCS]) and traditional dogs is the frequency of and age at initiation of periodontal care.

All canine patients should have homecare started at six months of age [7]. This is because it allows the client to "get ahead" of the disease as well as the fact that homecare training is easier to introduce in younger pets [8, 9]. However, it is more critical in "at risk" breeds to initiate homecare early. This is because they will develop gingivitis and attachment loss earlier, and that small breeds tend to be more resistant to homecare efforts.

10.1 Homecare

Homecare is a critical aspect of periodontal therapy [8]. The initial phase of plaque attachment is development of the pellicle on the surface of the teeth, which starts within *nanoseconds* of a prophylaxis [10]. True bacterial plaque will colonize clean tooth surfaces within 24 hours of cleaning [4, 11]. A recent study has shown that without homecare, bacterial counts return to pre-scaling levels in just one week [12]. It is well-established that without homecare, gingival infection and inflammation rapidly recur [13–17]. Finally, it was found in a human review that professional cleanings were of little value without homecare [18].

Homecare should be recommended to clients at the "well puppy" as well as all vaccine appointments. In addition, consider reinforcing the importance at the time of the spay/neuter surgery. Early onset homecare has the most effect as starting early might actually decrease the necessary frequency [19].

There are two major types of homecare: active (brushing and rinses) and passive (diets and chews).

Breed Predispositions to Dental and Oral Disease in Dogs, First Edition. Edited by Brook A. Niemiec.
© 2021 John Wiley & Sons, Inc. Published 2021 by John Wiley & Sons, Inc.

10.1.1 Active Homecare

- Active homecare is considered the "gold standard" of home dental care and should be recommended to all clients [20]. This technique has been shown to consistently and effectively decrease oral bacterial counts in dogs [21]. The only piece of equipment absolutely necessary is a tooth brush. There are numerous veterinary brushes available, and a proper brush should be selected based on patient size. Circular feline brushes[1] are effective products and should be considered along with the standard veterinary brushes.

  In addition to the veterinary products, human tooth brushes may be effective in animal patients. A soft bristled toothbrush is always recommended. A child's/infant's toothbrush is often the correct size for small and toy breed patients.

- **Pastes:** There are a plethora of veterinary toothpastes available, which greatly increase the acceptance of the toothbrush by the pet. In addition, they typically contain a calcium chelator[2] which has been shown to decrease the level of calculus deposits on the teeth [22, 23]. However, remember that calculus in and of itself is largely non-pathogenic [11]. The mechanical removal of plaque by the movement of the brush/instrument is the key to plaque control [20]. However, a recent study has shown that the paste itself also has some beneficial effects [12]. If the pet is resistant to brushing, this same study showed that application of the toothpaste has a positive effect.

  Palatability can also be improved by employing alternate flavorings [11, 24]. Tuna juice and beef broth are excellent products for increasing palatability and acceptance. This author recommends these options be used initially, and the additional benefits of the pastes be added once brushing is well tolerated by the patient. Human tooth pastes and products such as baking soda are *not* recommended as they contain detergents and/or fluoride which may cause gastric upset or event potentially fluorosis if swallowed [11, 24].

- **Antimicrobial preparations** are also available. These products further improve plaque and gingivitis control beyond that of pastes when combined with brushing. Therefore, they should potentially be prescribed instead of toothpaste in high-risk patients and in cases of established periodontal disease [25–27]. Chlorhexidine[3] has been shown in numerous studies to decrease gingivitis if applied consistently over time [28–30].

  Another effective oral antiseptic is soluble zinc salts, as they have been shown to decrease dental plaque [31]. One veterinary labeled oral zinc ascorbate gel[4] has been proven to decrease plaque and gingivitis [32], and provides the additional advantage of being tasteless (which should improve acceptance, especially in cats) [33]. This product also contains ascorbic acid which has been shown to support collagen synthesis [9, 34, 35], which may improve healing. Thus, application of this product post-operatively maintains the oral health until other forms of homecare can be instituted and improves healing.

- **Frequency:** Once a day is ideal, as this level of care is required to stay ahead of plaque formation [11, 16, 24, 36, 37]. In addition, every other day brushing has not been shown to be effective for gingivitis control [37]. Three days a week is generally accepted as the minimum frequency for patients *in good oral health* [19]. Once patients develop any level of periodontal disease (even just gingivitis), daily brushing is required to maintain oral health, and twice daily care may be necessary [16, 37–39]. Brushing once a week is insufficient to maintain oral health [36]. Finally, it should be noted that consistency with homecare is critical. If brushing is suspended for as little as

---

1 CET® Cat Toothbrush: Virbac animal health: Fort Worth TX.
2 Sodium hexametaphosphate.
3 Clensz-a-dent, Sogeval, Oldsmar, FL.
4 Maxiguard oral hygiene gel, Addison Biological Laboratory, Fayette, MO.

a month, the level of gingival inflammation will return to the same level as patients who received no therapy [40].

10.1.2 Passive Homecare

Since passive homecare requires no work by the owner, compliance is more likely. Compliance is especially important since long-term consistency is the key factor in the efficacy of home dental care [40]. It has been shown that the compliance rate with toothbrushing with *highly motivated* pet owners is only around 50% after six months [41]. In fact, one study showed that passive homecare may be superior to active homecare simply due to the fact that it is actually performed [42]. This should *not* be misconstrued to mean that it is more effective, just that the average client is poorly compliant.

The downfall of all chew-based passive homecare products involves the fact that pets typically do not chew with the entire mouth and therefore areas will be missed. Passive homecare is most effective on the carnassial and surrounding teeth, and in contrast, active homecare is superior for the incisor and canine teeth [43]. Therefore, a combination of active and passive homecare is best.

Passive homecare is an alternative for minimizing periodontal disease, and is achieved with special diets, chews and treats, as well as potentially water additives. Some of these methods are effective, but many are not. Some of the effective products are detailed below; however, there is not enough room here for a complete discussion of all products. The listed products are based on a thorough literature review as well as the author's extensive professional experience. It is recommended that the reader perform their own research and utilize the Veterinary Oral Health Council (VOHC®) to form proper client recommendations, rather than simply reading the marketing hype.

10.1.2.1 Diets for Dental Care

It has long been thought that standard dry dog food (kibble) supports oral health, with one study supporting these claims [44]. However, an additional paper confirmed that dry food was *not* superior to moist foods in regards to improving oral health [45]. However, there are several commercial diets available that have been shown to decrease plaque and/or tartar build-up [46]. These products employ abrasives to scrape plaque from the tooth surface. The individual kibbles of these specially formulated diets are generally larger than standard kibbles [22, 42]. This attribute increases the amount of chewing performed and thus improves the efficacy of the abrasive cleaning [47]. Many of the products also contain a calcium chelator[5] to further reduce dental calculus accumulation [22, 23, 48–50]. However, some studies have reported that it is the kibble size and not additives that improve oral health [51]. Also, as noted above, calculus is not a major player in the development of periodontal disease.

Several diets[6,7,8] have received the VOHC seal as effective in plaque and calculus reduction [52]. In addition, two additional diets[9,10] have received VOHC approval for calculus reduction only. One important point is that even though these products may decrease plaque and calculus, they are typically most effective on the areas around the cusp tips and not at the gingival margin [49]. Since supragingival plaque and calculus is essentially non-pathogenic, minimal medical benefit is achieved by these methods [53]. Of the available diets, only one[11] has been clinically proven to

---

5 Sodium hexametaphosphate.
6 Prescription diet t/d® Hills Pet Nutrition.
7 HealthyAdvantage™ Oral Care for: Hills Pet Nutrition.
8 Science Diet® Oral Care for Dogs: Hill's Pet Nutrition.
9 Eukanuba® Adult Maintenance Diet for Dogs: Iams: Dayton Ohio.
10 Purina Veterinary Diets® DH Dental Health™ brand canine and Feline Formulas: Purina Nestle Purina Petcare Company, St Louis, MO.
11 Prescription diet t/d Hills Pet Nutrition.

decrease gingivitis [54–56]. The main reason for this product's effectiveness lies in the diet's fiber arrangement. The alignment allows the tooth to fully pierce the kibble prior to it breaking apart, allowing the entire tooth (including the critical marginal area) to be cleaned.

10.1.2.2 Plaque and/or Calculus Control Treats

Plain baked biscuit treats and chew toys (e.g. string and rope toys) have not shown to be of benefit for the prevention of periodontitis [53]. However, there are numerous edible treats available for passive homecare, with varying efficacy.

The most common treats are rusks, products of compressed wheat or cellulose, and rawhide chews [50, 53, 57–60]. These products function similar to tartar control diets, with the abrasives cleaning the tooth surface, and may include calcium chelators or other substances to further increase their anti-plaque efficacy [61, 62]. However, as with the tartar control diets above, most of the beneficial effects are on the supragingival areas of the cheek teeth.

Of the numerous commercially available products, only a handful[12,13,14,15,16] have been clinically proven to decrease gingivitis [51, 58, 61, 63–67]. VOHC approval has been awarded to several of these products as well.[17,18,19,20,21,22,23,24]

The addition of chlorhexidine to rawhide chews[25] has shown benefit in the reduction of plaque in animal studies [68]. Another chew based treat[26] which also has VOHC approval and works well in this author's hands contains a different anti-plaque agent (delmopinol), which decreases plaque accumulation [69]. During chewing, these antiseptics are is spread throughout the mouth and may provide positive effects on these teeth. The delmopinol product also has a consistency which allows the teeth to chew through the entire treat, thus cleaning to the gingival margin.

A product containing the brown alga, *Ascophyllum nodosum*,[27] has been shown to improve oral health status [70]. This additive has also been incorporated into an edible treat which has VOHC approval.[28]

One important point to remember is that many chew treats which claim to help control dental disease are very hard in texture. The chewing of these products may (and often does) result in tooth fracture [71, 72]. A good rule of thumb is that if you cannot make an indentation into the product with your fingernail, it is too hard [20]. Also, just because a product is effective for dental disease, does not necessarily mean it is safe. Owners must be aware of the choking/obstructive possibilities of many treats. For this reason, the VOHC requires that products be safe to receive their seal of acceptance.

---

12 Greenies Dental Treats: Mars Petcare.
13 Pedigree Rask/Dentabone, Mars Petcare.
14 Tartar Shield Soft Rawhide Chews for Dogs Therametric Technologies, Inc.
15 Veggiedent: Virbac Animal Health.
16 CET hexachews®: Virbac Animal Health,
17 Hill's Science Diet Canine Oral Care Chews: Hills Pet Nutrition.
18 Purina Veterinary Diets Dental Chews brand Canine Treats: Purina.
19 Canine Greenies ® – all sizes and formulations: Mars Petcare.
20 Checkups Chews for Dogs, Diamond Foods Inc.
21 Veggiedent: Virbac Animal Health.
22 Purina DentaLife daily oral care dog treats: Nestle Purina.
23 Improved Milk-Bone Brushing Chews for Dogs: Big Heart Pet Brands.
24 VetIQ Minties Medium Dog Dental Treat: True RX.
25 CET hexachews: Virbac Animal Health.
26 Oravet dental hygiene chews: Boehringer–Ingelheim.
27 Plaque-off: Swedencare.
28 ProDen PlaqueOff Dental Bites: SwedenCare.

10.1.2.3 Water Additives

This is a relatively new area of home dental care, and there are several products available in this category. In general, this author does not recommend this class of passive homecare. However, one product[29] was shown to decrease plaque and calculus [73].

Conclusions

Homecare is an absolutely critical aspect of periodontal therapy, but it is widely ignored. Early and consistent client education is the key to compliance. There are numerous options available, but tooth brushing remains the gold standard. Of the numerous products available for passive homecare, only a few are truly effective, and the reader is urged to critically review the clinical studies when deciding which products to prescribe.

10.2 Professional Care

10.2.1 Professional dental cleaning

The foundation of in-clinic periodontal therapy is "Professional Dental Cleaning." While there are many names for this procedure (Complete Oral Health Assessment and Treatment (COHAT) and Oral Assessment, Treatment, and Prevention (ATP)), this is the current term recommended by the AVDC. These other terms serve to emphasize the fact that dental procedures in animals rarely are just "cleanings," and that the oral exam is an important aspect of the cleaning. Terms such as "dental" and "prophy" (prophylaxis) are no longer recommended as they do not accurately describe the procedure and therefore degrade the medical value of the procedure when properly executed. This is a medical procedure which must be performed meticulously to provide a medical benefit. There are various recipes for a complete dental cleaning, but this author recommends the following steps: [2]

1. Pre-anesthesia exam (oral and general physical) and work-up [79, 88]
   a. Qualify the patient for anesthesia
      i. Auscultation and pulse assessment (cardiovascular and respiratory)
      ii. Complete blood count (CBC), chemistry panel, urinalysis (UA; renal, liver, hemogram)
   b. Provide as accurate as possible estimate
      i. Time
      ii. Cost
2. Proper anesthesia and monitoring
   a. Decrease anesthesia morbidity and mortality [89]
   b. Remember most anesthetic deaths occur in recovery [90]
3. Chlorhexidine lavage
   a. Decrease bacterial load for patient and environment
4. Supragingival scaling
   a. Generally, with an ultrasonic scaler
5. Subgingival scaling
   a. **The most important step**
   b. Combination of hand and ultrasonic

---

29 Aquadent: Virbac animal health.

6. Polishing
   a. Smooth the tooth to retard future plaque attachment
7. Sulcal lavage
   a. Remove debris and decrease bacterial count
8. Oral exam and charting
   a. A combination of visual and tactile means
      i. Periodontal probing
      ii. Exploring
   b. Need a high-quality dental chart
9. Dental radiographs
   a. Critical for oral diagnosis and treatment [91–93]
10. Treatment planning and any additional therapy
   a. If a significant amount of work is necessary, staging is acceptable.
11. Application of a barrier sealant[30]
   a. This is an optional step for plaque control during the healing period.

Box 10.1 Initiation of Professional Care

Current recommendations for at-risk patients (dogs under 10 kg) is that the first dental procedure be performed at 9–12 months of age and then every 9–12 months [7]. Early intervention is important not only to perform a cleaning *before* dental disease starts, but also to evaluate for other pathologies which are common in small and at-risk dogs such as: impacted teeth, retained deciduous teeth, and mobile maxillary second premolars (see below for more information). Treating these conditions early will have a significant positive effect on the periodontal, maxillofacial, and overall health of these patients.

It is understood that this recommendation for early intervention is counter to what has been the standard of care in veterinary dentistry. Early adopters will likely face some to significant pushback from clients as well as colleagues. However, this is one of the most important parts of this text, which is to encourage proper *preventative* dental care for these at-risk breeds.

10.2.2 Additional Treatment Based on Exam and Dental Radiology

If there are no pockets greater than 3 mm, there is no minimal to no gingival recession, and no mobile teeth, the professional dental cleaning and homecare are sufficient. However, the vast majority of veterinary patients are not presented until advanced disease is present.

Pockets between 3 and 6-mm (Figure 10.1) without mobility or furcation exposure more than level 1 (Figure 10.2) can be treated with closed root planning +/− application of a perioceutic[31,32] [6, 94–98] (Figure 10.3). Any teeth with pockets over 6-mm (Figure 10.4), furcation level 2 or 3

---

30 Oravet Barrier Sealant. Boehringer–Ingelheim.
31 Clindorol.
32 Doxirobe.

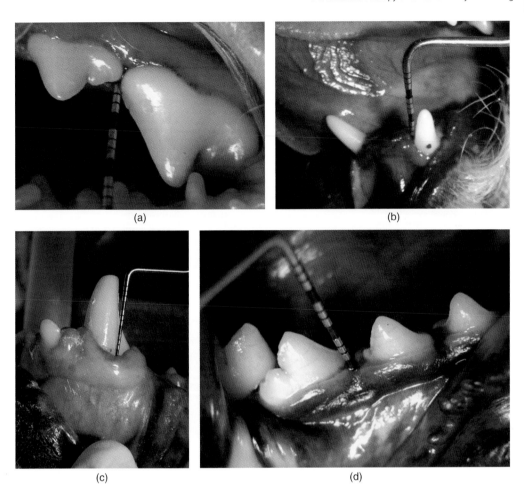

(a)   (b)

(c)   (d)

Figure 10.1 Pockets which can and should be treated with closed root planing. (a) Intraoral dental picture of the maxillary left premolars of a dog. There is a 5-mm pocket between the roots of the third and fourth premolar (207 and 208) without furcation exposure. The resulting loss is less than 50% and thus can be effectively cleaned with closed root planing. (b) Intraoral dental picture of the mandibular left canine (304) of a dog. There is a 5-mm pocket on the mesio-lingual aspect of the tooth. This can be effectively cleaned with closed root planing. (c) Intraoral dental picture of the mandibular left canine (304) of a dog. There is a 4-mm pocket on the buccal aspect of the tooth. This can be effectively cleaned with closed root planing. (d) Intraoral dental picture of the mandibular right premolars of a dog. There is a 4-mm pocket between the roots of the third and fourth premolar (407 and 408). The resulting loss is less than 50% and thus can be effectively cleaned with closed root planing.

(Figure 10.5), greater th-an 50% bone loss, (Figure 10.6) *or* are pathologically mobile require further therapy due to the inability to clean these areas without direct root visualization [96, 99, 100]. Note that any one of these findings necessitates advanced procedures. In small breed dogs, the best therapy is likely extraction as it is curative for the disease (at least for that tooth) [101]. However, if the client is interested in salvage, periodontal surgery +/− guided tissue regeneration can be performed [102, 103] (Figure 10.7). In these procedures, homecare and regular rechecks are necessary.

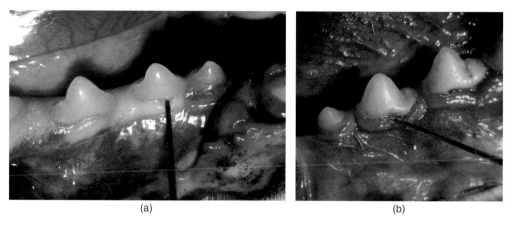

(a)   (b)

Figure 10.2 Class 1 furcation exposure on the buccal aspect of a mandibular right (a) and left (b) second premolar (406 and 306). These teeth can effectively be cleaned with closed root planing.

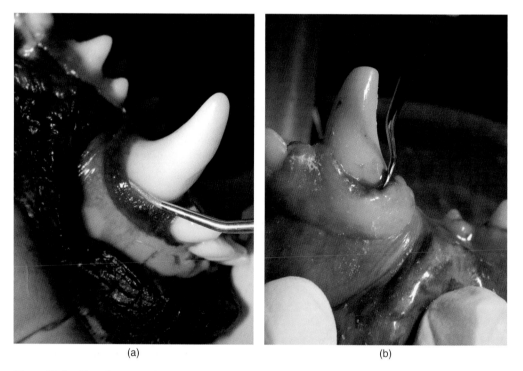

(a)   (b)

Figure 10.3 Closed root planing performed with a fine subgingival ultrasonic tip (a) and curette (b). Following the cleaning, perioceutic is applied to the pocket to help improve attachment gain (c).

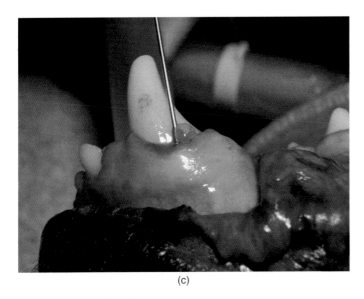

(c)

Figure 10.3 (*Continued*)

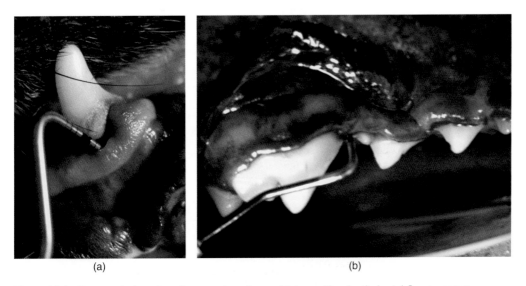

(a)   (b)

Figure 10.4 Deep periodontal pockets require advanced intervention (periodontal flap surgery or extraction) to reliably remove the infection. (a) A 13-mm periodontal pocket on the mesio-buccal aspect of the left mandibular canine (304). (b) A 15-mm periodontal pocket between the right maxillary third and fourth premolars (107 and 108). Both these teeth require extraction.

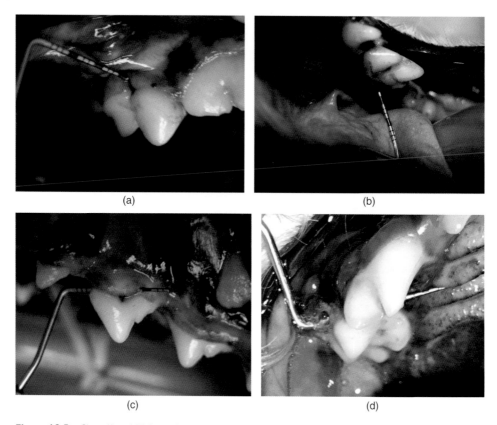

Figure 10.5 Class II and III furcation exposure requires periodontal flap surgery (ideally combined with guided tissue regeneration) or extraction to resolve the infection. (a) A class II furcation exposure on the buccal aspect of the right maxillary first molar (109). Either periodontal flap surgery or extraction is indicated. (b) A class II furcation exposure on the lingual aspect of the right mandibular first molar (409). Either periodontal flap surgery or extraction is indicated. Cases like this demonstrate the importance of a complete oral exam. (c) A class III furcation exposure on the left maxillary second premolar (206). Extraction of this tooth is indicated. (d) A class III furcation exposure on the right maxillary first molar (109). Extraction of this tooth is indicated.

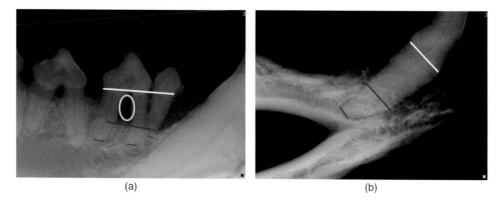

Figure 10.6 Dental radiographs of the right mandibular first and second premolar (405 and 406) (a) and canine (404) (b) demonstrating greater than 50% bone loss. The CEG (where the bone should be) is shown with a white line. The current level of bone is demonstrated by a red line. The apices are delimited by a purple line. Note that the second premolar in (a) also has class III furcation exposure (yellow circle). All of these teeth should be extracted.

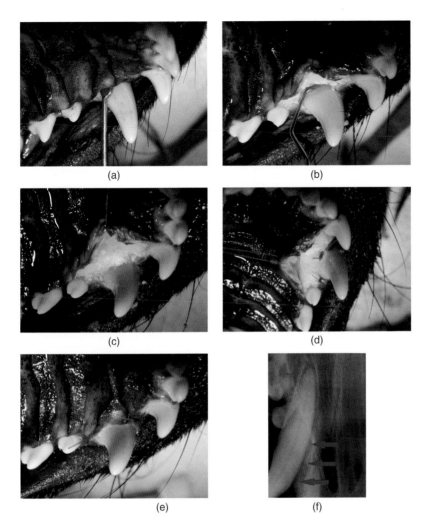

Figure 10.7 A brief example of the technique of guided tissue regeneration on the palatal surface of a maxillary canine. For more information and training on the procedure, the reader is directed to "Veterinary Periodontology" or better yet to a hands-on training session. To see the offerings by the author visit http://dogbeachvet.com. (a) An envelope flap is created on the palatal aspect of the tooth. (b) The exposed root surface is thoroughly cleaned with a combination of hand instrumentation (curettes) (pictured) and ultrasonic scalers. (c) Bone augmentation is placed in the cleaned defect. (d) A barrier membrane is placed over the bone augmentation. (e) The flap is replaced and sutured. As you can see, this technique is less invasive than an extraction, and allows the patient to maintain function of the tooth. (f) Pre-operative dental radiograph of the left maxillary canine in a patient with a deep vertical pocket on the palatine surface (red arrows). However, there is no current evidence of an ONF. This tooth was treated with a periodontal flap and guided tissue regeneration. The imaged premolars and third incisor were extracted due to periodontal disease. (g) Three year recheck radiograph of the patient in (f). Note that the bone on the palatal aspect has filled in very well (blue arrow). These teeth can be salvaged with appropriate therapy.

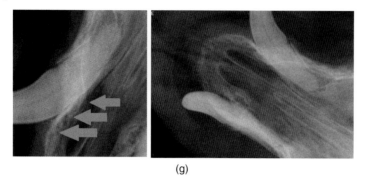

(g)

Figure 10.7 (*Continued*)

Box 10.2 The Case Against Anesthesia Free Dentistry

Any professional periodontal therapy for veterinary patients *must* be performed under general anesthesia, with a well-cuffed endotracheal tube [74–78]. Only when the patient is properly anesthetized can a safe and effective cleaning and oral evaluation be performed [79]. Despite its unfortunate popularity, non-anesthesia dentistry (NAD) provides no measurable medical benefit. A recent study revealed that patients who received this procedure actually had worse disease than those who did not [80] (Figure B10.1).

Other studies have proven that conscious exams greatly underestimate the true incidence and degree of periodontal disease [81, 82] (Figure B10.2). The increased difficulty in or performing conscious oral exams on small and toy breed dogs only serves to amplify this situation. The combination of insufficient cleaning (and a complete lack of subgingival treatment) and lack of quality oral exam (clinical and radiographic) results in a cosmetic benefit while leaving the patient to "suffer in silence" (Figure 10.10). Thus, the procedure typically provides a "false sense of security" as the teeth look clean, leading to significant delays in appropriate treatment.

The intensity of physical restraint required for these procedures and the resultant fear and anxiety cannot be dismissed. In addition, employing sharp instruments on the delicate gingival tissues as well as probing/exploring diseased teeth causes significant pain for the patient. Finally, substantial damage (to the patient and operator) can result if the patient suddenly moves (Figure B10.4). In short, the pain and anxiety elicited by this procedure without the administration of pain control and sedatives is simply unacceptable.

Finally, scaling has been shown to roughen the tooth surface (Figure B10.5), and that if the teeth are not effectively polished; plaque, calculus, and periodontal disease quickly recur [9, 11, 83–85]. This is yet another reason why this procedure is ineffective.

Based on the incontrovertible evidence above, numerous veterinary associations worldwide including essentially all veterinary dental groups, have position statements against its practice [86]. In fact, the World Small Animal Veterinary Association dental guidelines committee considers NAD an animal welfare concern [87]. Performing NAD is illegal in several states when performed outside of a veterinary practice. Finally, several governing bodies consider the practice below the standard of care.

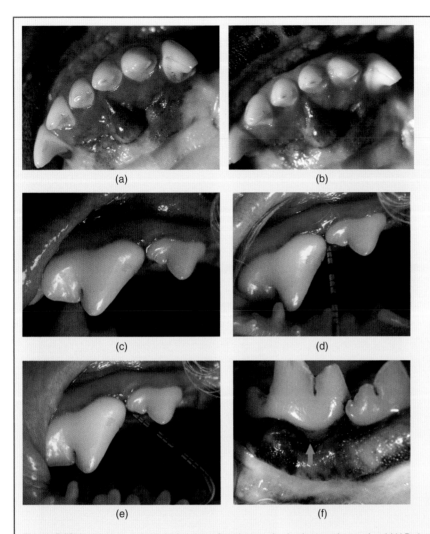

Figure B10.1 Intraoral dental pictures of patients who had recently received NAD. (a & b) A Shetland Sheepdog who received NAD regularly including just one week prior to presentation. (a) The palatal surface of the maxillary incisors. (b) The same area as in (a) following a professional dental scaling under general anesthesia. (c–e) A Chihuahua who had received NAD every other month for several years, who presented for "incisors falling out." On oral exam, the teeth were clean with no evidence of gingivitis, but there was an enamel defect on the fourth premolar. (c) However periodontal probing revealed a 5-mm periodontal pocket (d) as well as class II furcation exposure. (e) The NAD had produced clean crowns, but allowed for continued infection subgingivally. Luckily, this was caught in time and the tooth wasb saved with periodontal flap surgery and guided tissue regeneration. (f) Intraoral dental picture of a miniature poodle who had received regular NAD. The crowns were clean, but the roots were not. This allowed continued infection and subsequent attachment loss (blue arrow). (g) Intraoperative Intraoral dental picture of a French Bulldog who had received regular NAD. The crowns were clean, but the roots were not. This allowed continued infection and subsequent attachment loss (blue arrow). The second molar was extracted and the first molar treated with periodontal flap surgery and guided tissue regeneration.

(Continued)

Box 10.2 (Continued)

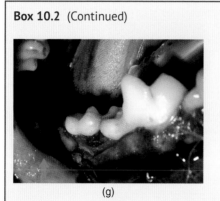

(g)

Figure B10.1 (*Continued*)

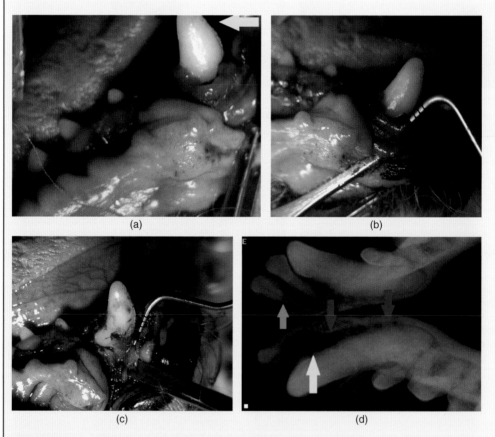

(a)   (b)

(c)   (d)

Figure B10.2 Intraoral dental picture of a canine patient had received NAD on a monthly basis (most recently two weeks prior) for three years. The patient was presented for persistent bad breath and was recommended by the NAD provider "to come every week for a while." (a) Evaluation under general anesthesia revealed the large amount of dental calculus on the lingual surface of the mandibular right canine (yellow arrow), whereas the remainder of the teeth looked clean. (b) Periodontal probing revealed the deep periodontal pocket on the lingual and facial surfaces of the teeth. (c) Following flap creation for surgical extraction, the subgingival dental calculus is evident. (d) Finally, the dental radiograph confirms the subgingival calculus (yellow arrow) and severe alveolar bone loss in the area (red arrows) predisposing the patient to a pathologic fracture. In addition, note the severe alveolar bone loss to the left incisors (blue arrow).

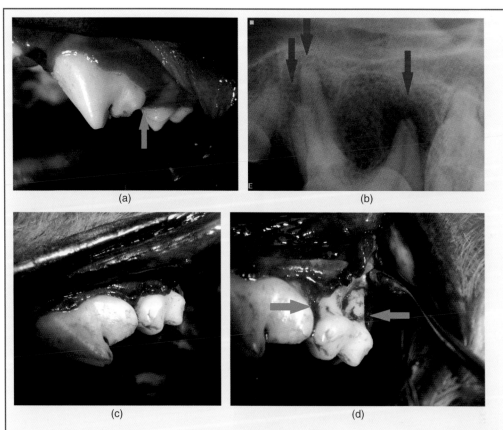

(a) (b)

(c) (d)

Figure B10.3 The lack of a quality oral exam in NAD allows for continued infection. (a) Intraoral picture of the maxillary left fourth premolar (208) of a Welsh Corgi presented for a carnassial abscess which had received NAD on a regular basis. Conscious oral exam by a Board-Certified Veterinary Dentist revealed the small fracture to the distal aspect of the tooth (blue arrow). (b) The intraoral dental radiograph revealed periapical rarefaction (red arrows) confirming the source of the infection. Note that infection is typically present for a lengthy period of time prior to creating a clinical abscess and that the imaged bone destruction is a lengthy process. Therefore, this infection has been present but undiagnosed for a long time. Proper oral care with a thorough oral exam and/or dental radiology would have allowed for much earlier treatment of this significant infection. (c) Intraoral picture of the maxillary left first molar (209) in a patient who recently received NAD. Note that the crowns of the teeth are very clean and there is no obvious evidence of gingivitis. (d) Intra-operative picture of the patient in (c). Note there is significant subgingival calculus and attachment loss (blue arrows). This tooth required extraction even though by outward appearance the tooth was healthy.

(Continued)

Box 10.2 (Continued)

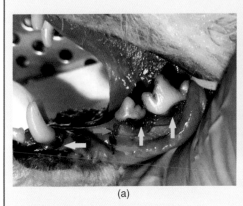
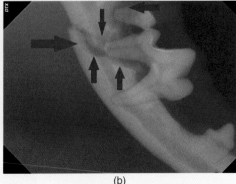

(a) (b)

Figure B10.4 (a) Intraoral dental picture of a Chihuahua who was presented on an emergency basis for a lacerated gingiva during a NAD (blue arrows). There was significant amount of periodontal disease also present due to the chronic ineffective therapy (yellow arrows). (b) Intraoral dental radiograph of the right mandible of a dog who had his jaw fractured during a non-anesthesia dentistry. There was significant bone loss from the chronic periodontal disease (purple arrows) that was not effectively treated and the jaw fractured (red arrow) during the restraint.

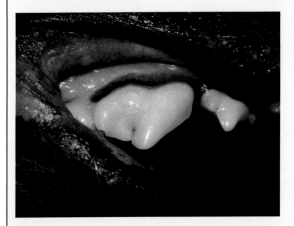

Figure B10.5 Right maxillary fourth premolar (108) of a patient who recently received NAD. Note the significant roughening of the enamel. This will create much faster plaque accumulation and hasten periodontal disease recurrence.

10.2.3 Plaque Control During the Healing Period

Currently, the majority of small breed dogs presented for dental therapy require some form of surgical correction (generally extractions). Therefore, quite often suturing has been performed and healing time is required. In general, veterinary dentists recommend two weeks of soft food and no brushing to allow for the tissues to fully heal. However, as we know, in just two weeks, plaque and calculus have already populated the tooth surface, and gingivitis may be present. This leads to a common question among clients and veterinary professionals, "How do we keep the teeth clean during this time?"

In this author's opinion, there are a few effective and economical ways to "bridge" the time between surgery and the institution of traditional homecare methods. The preferred method in this author's practices is the application of a wax-based barrier sealant[33] [104]. This product has been shown to effectively resist plaque attachment for two weeks following application. Another advantage is that the client does not need to manipulate the patient's mouth during the healing period.

The other option is application of antiseptic rinses and gels. Chlorhexidine products are well-known to decrease plaque and gingivitis when applied daily to the dentition. In addition, an oral zinc ascorbate gel[34] has been proven to decrease plaque and gingivitis as well as support collagen synthesis, which may improve healing. (See antimicrobial preparations above for a more complete discussion of these products.) After healing has occurred, tooth brushing or an effective form of passive homecare can be instituted. Alternatively, antiseptics and/or a weekly application of the barrier sealant can be continued or added to these other methods.

Editor's note: This was a brief synopsis of periodontal therapy and mostly specific to small breed dogs. Practitioners should not rely on this text as sufficient for a complete understanding of periodontal disease. For more information on this disease process and its treatment the reader is directed to the Wiley text "Veterinary Periodontology" by Dr. Brook Niemiec.

References

1 Niemiec, B.A. (2012). Etiology and pathogenesis of periodontal disease. In: *Veterinary Periodontology* (ed. B.A. Niemiec), 18–32. Ames: Wiley.

2 Niemiec, B.A. (2013). The complete dental cleaning. In: *Veterinary Periodontology* (ed. B.A. Niemiec), 129–153. Ames: Wiley Blackwell.

3 Lindhe, J., Hamp, S., and Löe, H. (1975). Plaque induced periodontal disease in beagle dogs: a 4-year clinical, roentgenographical and histometrical study. *J. Periodontal Res.* 10: 243–255.

4 Boyce, E.N., Ching, R.J., Logan, E.I. et al. (1995). Occurrence of Gram-negative black-pigmented anaerobes in subgingival plaque during the development of canine periodontal disease. *Clin. Infect. Dis.* 20 (Suppl. 2): S317–S319.

5 Loe, H., Theilade, E., and Jensen, S.B. (1965). Experimental gingivitis in man. *J. Periodontol.* 36: 177.

6 Niemiec, B.A. (2012). Advanced non-surgical therapy. In: *Veterinary Periodontology* (ed. B.A. Niemiec), 154–169. Ames: Wiley.

7 Bellows, J., Berg, M.L., Dennis, S. et al. (2019, 2019). AAHA dental care guidelines for dogs and cats. *J. Am. Anim. Hosp. Assoc.* 55 (2): 49–69.

8 Niemiec, B.A. (2012). Home plaque control. In: *Veterinary Periodontology* (ed. B.A. Niemiec), 175–185. Ames: Wiley-Blackwell.

9 Holmstrom, S.E., Frost, P., and Eisner, E.R. (1998). Dental prophylaxis. In: *Veterinary Dental Techniques*, 2e, 133–166. Philadelphia, PA: Saunders.

10 Quirynen, M., Teughels, W., Kinder Haake, S., and Newman, M.G. (2006). *Microbiology of Periodontal Diseases, in: Carranza's Clinical Periodontology*, 134–169. St. Louis, Mo: WB Saunders.

---

33 Oravet Barrier Sealant BI.
34 Maxiguard Oral Hygiene Gel, Addison Biological Laboratory, Fayette, MO.

11 Wiggs, R.B. and Lobprise, H.B. (1997). Periodontology. In: *Veterinary Dentistry, Principals and Practice*, 186–231. Philadelphia, PA: Lippincott-Raven.

12 Watanabe, K., Kijima, S., Nonaka, C. et al. (2016). Inhibitory effect for proliferation of oral bacteria in dogs by tooth brushing and application of toothpaste. *J. Vet. Med. Sci.* 78 (7): 1205–1208.

13 Debowes, L.J. (2010). Problems with the gingiva. In: *Small Animal Dental, Oral and Maxillofacial Disease, a Color Handbook* (ed. B.A. Niemiec), 159–181. London: Manson.

14 Fiorellini, J.P., Ishikawa, S.O., and Kim, D.M. (2006). *Clinical Features of Gingivitis, in: Carranza's Clinical Periodontology*, 362–372. St. Louis, MO: WB Saunders.

15 Rober, M. (2007). Effect of scaling and root planing without dental homecare on the subgingival microbiota. In: *Proceedings of the 16th European Congress of Veterinary Dentistry*, 28–30.

16 Corba, N.H., Jansen, J., and Pilot, T. (1986). Artificial periodontal defects and frequency of tooth brushing in beagle dogs (II). Clinical findings after a period of healing. *J. Clin. Periodontol.* 13 (3): 186–189.

17 Payne, W.A., Page, R.C., Olgolvie, A.L. et al. (1975). Histopathologic features of the initial and early stages of experimental gingivitis in man. *J. Periodontal Res.* 10: 51.

18 Needleman, I., Suvan, J., Moles, D.R., and Pimlott, J. (2005). A systematic review of professional mechanical plaque removal for prevention of periodontal diseases. *J. Clin. Periodontol.* 32 (Suppl. 6): 229–282.

19 Tromp, J.A., Jansen, J., and Pilot, T. (1986 Feb). Gingival health and frequency of tooth brushing in the beagle dog model. Clinical findings. *J. Clin. Periodontol.* 13 (2): 164–168.

20 Hale, F.A. (2003). Home care for the veterinary dental patient. *J. Vet. Dent.* 20 (1): 52–54.

21 Watanabe, K., Hayashi, K., Kijima, S. et al. (2015 Oct). Tooth brushing inhibits oral bacteria in dogs. *J. Vet. Med. Sci.* 77 (10): 1323–1325.

22 Hennet, P., Servet, E., Soulard, Y., and Biourge, V. (2007 Dec). Effect of pellet food size and polyphosphates in preventing calculus accumulation in dogs. *J. Vet. Dent.* 24 (4): 236–239.

23 Liu, H., Segreto, V.A., Baker, R.A. et al. (2002). Anticalculus efficacy and safety of a novel whitening dentifrice containing sodium hexametaphosphate: a controlled six-month clinical trial. *J. Clin. Dent.* 13 (1): 25–28.

24 Niemiec, B.A. (2008). Periodontal disease. *Top. Companion Anim. Med.* 23 (2): 72–80.

25 Stratul, S.I., Rusu, D., Didilescu, A. et al. (2010 Feb). Prospective clinical study evaluating the long-time adjunctive use of chlorhexidine after one-stage full-mouth SRP. *Int. J. Dent. Hyg.* 8 (1): 35–40.

26 Eaton, K.A., Rimini, F.M., Zak, E. et al. (1997). The effects of a 0.12% chlorhexidine-digluconate containing mouthrinse versus a placebo on plauq and gingival inflammation over a 3-month period. A multicentre study carried out in general dental practices. *J. Clin. Periodontol.* 24 (3): 189–197.

27 Hennet, P. (2002). Effectiveness of a dental gel to reduce plaque in beagle dogs. *J. Vet. Dent.* 19 (1): 11–14.

28 Hamp, S.E. and Emilson, C.G. (1973). Some effects of chlorhexidine on the plaque flora of the beagle dog. *J. Periodontol Res.* 12: 28–35.

29 Hull, P.S. and Davies, R.M. (1972). The effect of a chlorhexidine gel on tooth deposits in beagle dogs. *J. Small Anim. Pract.* 13: 207–212.

30 Maruniak, J., Clark, W.B., Walker, C.B. et al. (1992 Jan). The effect of 3 mouthrinses on plaque and gingivitis development. *J. Clin. Periodontol.* 19 (1): 19–23.

31 Wolinsky, L.E., Cuomo, J., Quesada, K. et al. (2000). A comparative pilot study of the effects of a dentifrice containing green tea bioflavonids, sanguinarine, or triclosan on oral bacterial biofilm formation. *J. Clin. Dent.* 11: 535–559.

32 Clarke, D.E. (2001). Clinical and microbiological effects of oral zinc ascorbate gel in cats. *J. Vet. Dent.* 18 (4): 177–183.

33 Niemiec, B.A. (2013). Home Plaque Control. In: *Veterinary Periodontology*, 75–86. Ames: Wiley-Blackwell.

34 Pinnel, S.R., Murad, S., and Darr, D. (1987). Induction of collagen synthesis by ascorbic acid. A possible mechanism. *Arch. Dermatol.* 123 (12): 1684–1686.

35 Murad, S., Grove, D., Lindberg, K.A. et al. (1981). Regulation of collagen synthesis by ascorbic acid. *Proc. Natl. Acad. Sci. USA.* 78 (5): 2879–2882.

36 Harvey, C., Serfilippi, L., and Barnvos, D. (2015 Spring). Effect of frequency of brushing teeth on plaque and calculus accumulation, and gingivitis in dogs. *J. Vet. Dent.* 32 (1): 16–21.

37 Gorrel, C. and Rawlings, J.M. (1996). The role of tooth-brushing and diet in the maintenance of periodontal health in dogs. *J. Vet. Dent.* 13 (4): 139–143.

38 Corba, N.H., Jansen, J., and Pilot, T. (1986). Artificial periodontal defects and frequency of tooth brushing in beagle dogs (I). Clinical findings after a period of healing. *J. Clin. Periodontol.* 13 (3): 158–163.

39 Tromp, J.A., van Rijn, L.J., and Jansen, J. (1986). Experimental gingivitis and frequency of tooth brushing in the beagle dog . Clinical findings. *J. Clin. Periodontol.* 13 (3): 190–194.

40 Ingham, K.E. and Gorrel, C. (2001). Effect of long-term intermittent periodontal care on canine periodontal disease. *J. Small Anim. Pract.* 42 (2): 67–70.

41 Miller, B.R. and Harvey, C.E. (1994). Compliance with oral hygiene recommendations following periodontal treatment in client-owned dogs. *J. Vet. Dent.* 11 (1): 18–19.

42 Vrieling, H.E., Theyse, L.F., van Winkelhoff, A.J. et al. (2005). Effectiveness of feeding large kibbles with mechanical cleaning properties in cats with gingivitis. *Tijdschr. Diergeneeskd.* 130 (5): 136–140.

43 Capik, I. (2007). Periodontal health vs. different preventive means in toy breeds – clinical study. In: *Proceedings of the 16th European Congress of Veterinary Dentistry*, 31–34.

44 Gawor, J.P., Reiter, A.M., Jodkowska, K. et al. (2006). Influence of diet on oral health in cats and dogs. *J. Nutr.* 136: 2021–23S.

45 Harvey, C.E., Shofer, F.S., and Laster, L. (1996). Correlation of diet, other chewing activities, and periodontal disease in north American client-owned dogs. *J. Vet. Dent.* 13: 101–105.

46 Jensen, L., Logan, E., Finney, O. et al. (1995). Reduction in accumulation of plaque, stain, and calculus in dogs by dietary means. *J. Vet. Dent.* 12 (4): 161–163.

47 Larsen, J. (2010). Oral products and dental disease. *Compend. Contin. Educ. Vet.* 32: E1–E3.

48 White, D.J., Cox, E.R., Suszcynskymeister, E.M., and Baig, A.A. (2002). In vitro studies of the anticalculus efficacy of a sodium hexametaphosphate whitening dentifrice. *J. Clin. Dent.* 13 (1): 33–37.

49 Stookey, G.K. and Warrick, J.M. (2005). Calculus prevention in dogs provided diets coated with HMP. In: *Proceedings of the 19th Annual American Veterinary Dental Forum*, 417–421. Orlando.

50 Lage, A., Lausen, N., Tracy, R., and Allred, E. (1990). Effect of chewing rawhide and cereal biscuit on removal of dental calculus in dogs. *JAVMA* 197 (2): 213–219.

51 Brown, W.Y. and McGenity, P. (2005). Effective periodontal disease control using dental hygiene chews. *J. Vet. Dent.* 22 (1): 16–19.

52 Veterinary Oral Health Council (2018). Diets and products for plaque and calculus reduction. www.vohc.org (accessed 27 June 2020).

53 Roudebush, P., Logan, E., and Hale, F.A. (2005). Evidence-based veterinary dentistry: a systematic review of homecare for prevention of periodontal disease in dogs and cats. *J. Vet. Dent.* 22 (1): 6–15.

54 Logan, E.I., Finney, O., and Hefferren, J.J. (2002). Effects of a dental food on plaque accumulation and gingival health in dogs. *J. Vet. Dent.* 19 (1): 15–18.

55 Logan, E.I., Proctor, V., Berg, M.L. et al. (2001). Dietary effect on tooth surface debris and gingival health in cats. In: *Proceedings of the 15th Annual American Veterinary Dental Forum*, 377. San Antonio.

56 Logan, E.I., Berg, M.L., Coffman, L. et al. (1999). Dietary control of feline gingivitis: results of a six month study. In: *Proceedings of the 13th Veterinary Dental Forum*, 54.

57 Hennet, P., Servet, E., and Venet, C. (2006). Effectiveness of an oral hygiene chew to reduce dental deposits in small breed dogs. *J. Vet. Dent.* 23 (1): 6–12.

58 Stookey, G.K. (2009). Soft rawhide reduces calculus formation in dogs. *J. Vet. Dent.* 26: 82–85.

59 Hennet, P. (2001). Effectiveness of an enzymatic rawhide dental chew to reduce plaque in beagle dogs. *J. Vet. Dent.* 18: 61–64.

60 Beynen, A.C., Van Altena, F., and Visser, E.A. (2010). Beneficial effect of a cellulose-containing chew treat on canine periodontal disease in a double-blind, placebo-controlled trial. *Am. J. Anim. Vet. Sci.* 5: 192–195.

61 Warrick, J.M., Stookey, G.K., Inskeep, G.A., and Inskeep, T.K. (2001). Reducing caclculus accumulation in dogs using an innovative rawhide treat system coated with hexametaphosphate. In: *Proceedings of the 15th Annual American Veterinary Dental Forum*, 379–382. San Antonio.

62 Stookey, G.K., Warrick, J.M., and Miller, L.L. (1995). Effect of sodium hexametaphosphate on dental calculus formation in dogs. *Am. J. Vet. Res.* 56: 913–918.

63 Gorrel, C. and Bierer, T.L. (1999). Long-term effects of a dental hygiene chew on the periodontal health of dogs. *J. Vet. Dent.* 16 (3): 109–113.

64 Gorrel, C., Warrick, J., and Bierer, T.L. (1999). Effect of a new dental hygiene chew on periodontal health in dogs. *J. Vet. Dent.* 16 (2): 77–81.

65 Mariani, C., Douhain, J., Servet, E. et al. (2009). Effect of toothbrushing and chew distribution on halitosis in dogs. In: *Proceedings of the 18th Congress of Veterinary Dentistry*, 13–15. Zurich.

66 Quest, B.W. (2013). Oral health benefits of a daily dental chew in dogs. *J. Vet. Dent.* 30: 84–87.

67 Clarke, D.E., Kelman, M., and Perkins, N. (2011). Effectiveness of a vegetable dental chew on periodontal disease parameters in toy breed dogs. *J. Vet. Dent.* 28: 230–235.

68 Rawlings, J.M., Gorrel, C., and Markwell, P.J. (1998). Effect on canine oral health of adding chlorhexidine to a dental hygiene chew. *J. Vet. Dent.* 15: 129–134.

69 Claydon, N., Hunter, L., Moran, J. et al. (1996). A 6-month home-usage trial of 0.1% and 0.2% delmopinol mouthwashes (I). Effects on plaque, gingivitis, supragingival calculus and tooth staining. *J. Clin. Periodontol.* 23 (3 Pt 1): 220–228.

70 Gawor, J., Jank, M., Jodkowska, K. et al. (2018). Effects of edible treats containing *Ascophyllum nodosum* on the Oral health of dogs: a double-blind, randomized, placebo-controlled single-Center study. *Front. Vet. Sci.* 5: 168.

71 Soltero-Rivera, M., Elliott, M.I., Hast, M.W. et al. (2019). Fracture limits of maxillary fourth premolar teeth in domestic dogs under applied forces. *Front Vet. Sci.* 5: 339.

72 British Veterinary Dental Association Position Statements (2019). www.bvda.co.uk/position-statements (accessed 27 June 2020).

73 Clarke, D.E. (2006). Drinking water additive decreases plaque and calculus accumulation in cats. *J. Vet. Dent.* 23: 79–82.

74 Colmery, B. (2005). The gold standard of veterinary oral health care. *Vet. Clin. North Am.* 35 (4): 781–787.

75 Niemiec, B.A. (2003). Professional teeth cleaning. *J. Vet. Dent.* 20 (3): 175–180.

76 Bellows, J. (2004). Equipping the dental practice. In: small animal dental equipment, materials, and techniques, a primer. *Blackwell*: 13–55.

77 Holmstrolm, S.E., Frost, P., and Eisner, E.R. (2002). Dental prophylaxis and periodontal disease stages. In: *Veterinary Dental Techniques*, 3e, 175–232. Philadelphia, PA: Saunders.

78 Holmstrom, S.E., Bellows, J., Juriga, S. et al. (2013). American Veterinary Dental College. 2013 AAHA Dental Care Guidelines for Dogs and Cats. *J. Am. Anim. Hosp. Assoc.* 49 (2): 75–82.

79 Huffman, L.J. (2010). Oral examination. In: *Small Animal Dental, Oral and Maxillofacial Disease, a Color Handbook* (ed. B.A. Niemiec), 39–61. London: Manson.

80 Urfer, S.R., Wang, M., Yang, M. et al. (2019). Risk factors associated with lifespan in pet dogs evaluated in primary care veterinary hospitals. *J. Am. Anim. Hosp. Assoc.* 55 (3): 130–137.

81 Bauer, A.E., Stella, J., Lemmons, M., and Croney, C.C. (2018). Evaluating the validity and reliability of a visual dental scale for detection of periodontal disease (PD) in non-anesthetized dogs (Canis familiaris). *PLoS One* 13 (9): e0203930.

82 Wallis, C., Patel, K.V., Marshall, M. et al. (2018). *J. Small Anim. Pract.* 59 (9): 560–569.

83 Bellows, J. (2004). Periodontal equipment, materials, and techniques. In: *Small Animal Dental Equipment, Materials, and Techniques, a Primer*, 115–173. Blackwell.

84 Silness, J. (1980). Fixed prosthodontics and periodontal health. *Dent. Clin. N. Am.* 24 (2): 317–329.

85 Berglundh, T., Gotfredsen, K., Zitzmann, N.U. et al. (2007). Spontaneous progression of ligature induced peri-implantitis at implants with different surface roughness: an experimental study in dogs. *Clin. Oral Implants Res.* 18 (5): 655–661.

86 AVDC position statement against NAD. (2018). http://AVDC.org (accessed 27 June 2020).

87 World Small Animal Veterinary Association Dental Guidelines Committee (2018). NAD is an animal welfare concern. http://Wsava.org (accessed 27 June 2020).

88 Joubert, K.E. (2007 Mar). Pre-anesthetic screening of geriatric dogs. *J. S. Afr. Vet. Assoc.* 78 (1): 31–35.

89 Brodbelt, D.C., Pfeiffer, D.U., Young, L.E. et al. (2007). Risk factors for anaesthetic-related death in cats: results from the confidential enquiry into perioperative small animal fatalities (CEPSAF). *Br. J. Anaesth.* 99: 617–623.

90 Brodbelt, D.C., Blissitt, K.J., Hammond, R.A. et al. (2008). The risk of death: the confidential enquiry into perioperative small animal fatalities. *Vet. Anaesth. Analg.* 35: 365–373.

91 Verstraete, F.J., Kass, P.H., and Terpak, C.H. (1998). Diagnostic value of full-mouth radiography in cats. *Am. J. Vet. Res.* 59 (6): 692–695.

92 Verstraete, F.J., Kass, P.H., and Terpak, C.H. (1998). Diagnostic value of full-mouth radiography in dogs. *Am. J. Vet. Res.* 59 (6): 686–691.

93 Niemiec, B.A. (2011). The importance of dental radiology. *Euro. J. Companion Anim.Pract.* 20: 219–229.

94 Gulati, M., Anand, V., Govila, V., and Jain, N. (2014). Host modulation therapy: an indispensable part of perioceutics. *J. Indian Soc. Periodontol.* 18 (3): 282–288.

95 Mahajania, M., Laddha, R., Shelke, A. et al. (2018). Effect of subgingival doxycycline placement on clinical and microbiological parameters in inflammatory periodontal disease: both in vivo and in vitro studies. *J. Contemp. Dent. Pract.* 19 (10): 1228–1234.

96 Zetner, K. and Rothmueller, G. (2002). Treatment of periodontal pockets with doxycycline in beagles. *Vet. Ther.* 3 (4): 441–452.

97 Jeffcoat, M.K., Bray, K.S., Ciancio, S.G. et al. (1998). Adjunctive use of a subgingival controlled-release chlorhexidine chip reduces probing depth and improves attachment level compared with scaling and root planing alone. *J. Periodontol.* 69 (9): 989–997.

98 Martel, D.P., Fox, P.R., Lamb, K.E., and Carmichael, D.T. (2019). Comparison of closed root planing with versus without concurrent doxycycline hyclate or clindamycin hydrochloride gel application for the treatment of periodontal disease in dogs. *J. Am. Vet. Med. Assoc.* 254 (3): 373–379.

99 Caffesse, R.G., Sweeney, P.L., and Smith, B.A. (1986). Scaling and root planing with and without periodontal flap surgery. *J. Clin. Periodontol.* 13 (3): 205–210.

100 Carranza, F.A. and Takei, H.H. (2006). *Phase II Periodontal Therapy, in Carranza's Clinical Periodontology*, 881–886. St. Louis, MO: WB Saunders.

101 Danser, M.M., van Winklehoff, A.J., de Graff, J. et al. (1994). Short term effect of full mouth extraction on periodontal pathogens colonizing the oral mucous membranes. *J. Clin. Periodontol.* 21: 484.

102 Niemiec, B.A. (2012). Periodontal flap surgery. In: *Veterinary Periodontology* (ed. B.A. Niemiec), 206–248. Ames: Wiley-Blackwell.

103 Niemiec, B.A. (2012). Osseous surgery and guided tissue regeneration. In: *Veterinary Periodontology* (ed. B.A. Niemiec), 254–288. Ames: Wiley-Blackwell.

104 Gengler, W.R., Kunkle, B.N., Romano, D. et al. (2005). Evaluation of a barrier sealant in dogs. *J. Vet. Dent.* 22: 157–159.

11

The Unique Challenges of Extractions in Small and Toy Breed Dogs

Brook A. Niemiec

Veterinary Dental Specialties and Oral Surgery, San Diego, CA, USA

Extractions must be undertaken with great care in small and toy breed dogs for several reasons. First, their jaws are much smaller and therefore more fragile than larger breeds [1]. Next, their teeth are proportionally larger, especially the mandibular first molar [2] (Figure 11.1). Furthermore, mandibular canines make up approximately 60–70% of the mandible [3] (Figure 11.2). This makes idiopathic mandibular fractures during extractions much more likely [4]. The fact that these patients also tend to have advanced periodontal disease, thus weakening the fragile bone, further increases the fracture risk [1, 5–9].

The increased root length in small and toy breed dogs also places the roots near the mandibular canal and nasal cavity. In some cases, the apex resides within the mandibular canal and occasionally runs all the way through it to the ventral cortex (Figure 11.3a). This situation creates two additional concerns which are unique to small breeds. First, there is the chance of injuring the mandibular nerve and artery during the extraction. This most often occurs with elevators, but can be much more damaging in cases where the bone must be removed to the level of the mandibular canal due to ankylosis (Figure 11.3b). The other concern when the apices are close/in the mandibular canal/nasal cavity, is breaking and/or forcing a root in the mandibular canal or nasal cavity (Figure 11.4). This often results because of ankyloses, and leads to attempting to extract a retained tooth root blind. Whenever a root breaks, a surgical extraction with visualization of the root remnant is always recommended [10] (Figure 11.5). In these cases (especially if the root lies near or in the nasal cavity or canal), referral to a veterinary dentist is advised.

Breed Predispositions to Dental and Oral Disease in Dogs, First Edition. Edited by Brook A. Niemiec.
© 2021 John Wiley & Sons, Inc. Published 2021 by John Wiley & Sons, Inc.

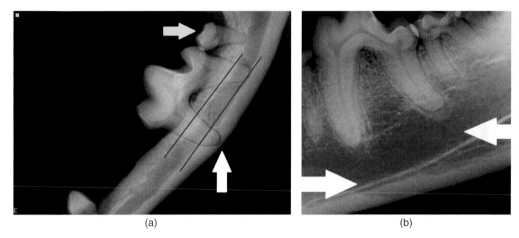

(a)   (b)

Figure 11.1 Comparison of the distal mandible in small and large breed dogs. (a) Intraoral dental radiograph of the mandibular molar in a 1.2-kg, nine-year-old dog. The mesial root naturally extends to within 0.4 mm of the ventral cortex (white arrow). This greatly increases the chances of an iatrogenic fracture occurring during the extraction attempt. This would be worsened in cases of advanced periodontal disease. Further, the roots of this tooth reside in the mandibular canal (red lines). The owner must be warned of the possibility of mandibular fracture and referral is recommended in these situations. Finally, note the periodontal loss on the second molar (yellow arrow). (b) Intraoral dental radiograph of the distal mandible of a 39 kg, eight-year-old dog. The apices of the first molar end over 2.5 cm from the ventral cortex (white arrows). This means that even if the tooth had complete periodontal loss, there would be plenty of bone remaining to effectively resist fracture.

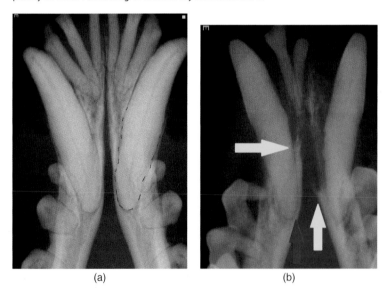

(a)   (b)

Figure 11.2 Radiographs demonstrating the minimal amount of bone surrounding the mandibular canines in small breed dogs. (a) Intraoral dental radiograph of the normal rostral mandible of a 3-kg five-year-old dog. The root takes up the vast majority of the bone in the area (dashed red line). The minimal bone greatly increases the chances of an iatrogenic fracture occurring during the extraction attempt. This is worsened in cases of advanced periodontal disease (see b). The owner must be warned of the possibility of mandibular fracture and referral is recommended for these extractions. (b) Intraoral dental radiograph of the rostral mandible of a 4-kg nine-year-old dog with advanced periodontal disease (yellow arrows). The bone loss in combination with the minimal natural bone (red arrow) further increases the chances of an iatrogenic fracture occurring during the extraction attempt. The owner must be warned of the possibility of mandibular fracture and referral is recommended in these situations.

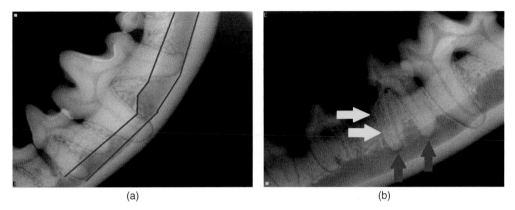

(a) (b)

Figure 11.3 (a) Intraoral dental radiograph of the distal mandible of a 2.2 kg eight-year-old dog. The roots of this tooth reside in the mandibular canal (red lines). Therefore, extreme care must be taken not to damage the delicate neurovascular structures which reside there. Also, hemostatic agents should always be prepared *prior* to the extraction. (b) Intraoral dental radiograph of the distal mandible of a 2.1 kg seven-year-old dog. The roots of the fourth premolar reside in the mandibular canal (red arrows). In addition, there is significant ankylosis and resorption, particularly to the mesial root (yellow arrows). Therefore, significant bone will need to be removed in order to extract the tooth, further increasing the chances of mandibular fracture. Also, bone removal to the level of the mandibular canal is likely required, thus risking damage to the neurovascular bundle. As above, care and preparation as well as informed consent is critical in these cases.

The fact that the roots are relatively larger, creates an additional issue with spacing. The apices of the mandibular teeth commonly have curves which are not commonly seen in large breed dogs (Figure 11.6). These curves can significantly increase the chance for iatrogenic issues such as root and jaw fracture [10, 11].

The smaller jaw will often result in invergent or fused roots (Figure 11.7). This will complicate extractions by changing the angle. And perhaps more importantly, it is important to know that the tooth does not require sectioning.

Finally, the small size of the facial structures places the globe very close to the apices of the molars and distal root of the fourth premolar. Severe iatrogenic eye traumas can occur during extraction attempts of maxillary molars if care is not taken, which may result in loss of the eye [12] (Figure 11.8).

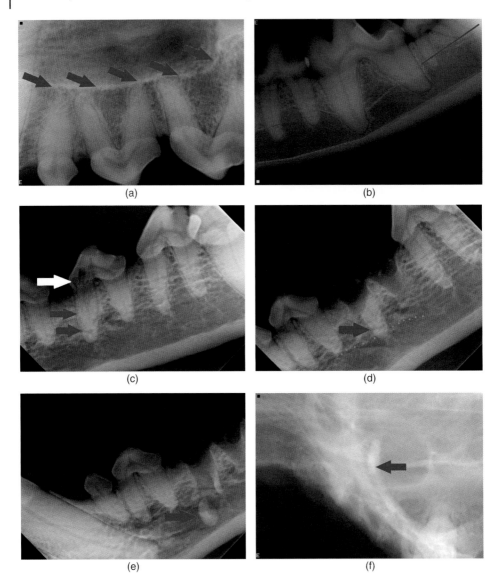

Figure 11.4 Roots in the mandibular canal or nasal cavity. (a) Normal intraoral dental radiograph of the maxillary first through third premolars in a 3 kg, six-year-old dog. The radiodense white line (palatine process of the maxilla, red arrows) is the transition between maxillary bone and the nasal cavity. The roots extend to within 1 m of the nose, thus risking displacement of the roots into the nasal cavity if care is not taken, especially with apical periodontitis. (b) Normal intraoral dental radiograph of the mandibular fourth premolar through second molar in a 1.5 kg, four-year-old dog. All imaged roots extend to reside within the mandibular canal (red lines), thus creating a significant risk of displacement of the roots into the canal if care is not taken. (c) Pre-operative intraoral dental radiograph of the mandibular left in a 4 kg, 12 year old dog with advanced tooth resorption on the second premolar (white arrow). The tooth resorption has resulted in significant ankylosis of the mesial root (red arrows). (d) Intraoperative dental radiograph of the tooth in (c). The resorption and ankylosis resulted in a fractured and retained root (red arrow) lying just inside the mandibular canal (dorsal aspect delineated by a dashed blue line). (e) Post-operative dental radiograph of the patient in (c and d) revealing that the root has been forced into the mandibular canal (red arrow). This occurred because the veterinarian attempted to elevate the root "blind" and thus was not elevating in the periodontal ligament space, rather pushing on the root itself. The patient was referred to a specialist for removal. (f) Palatine root of the left maxillary fourth premolar displaced into the nasal cavity (red arrow).

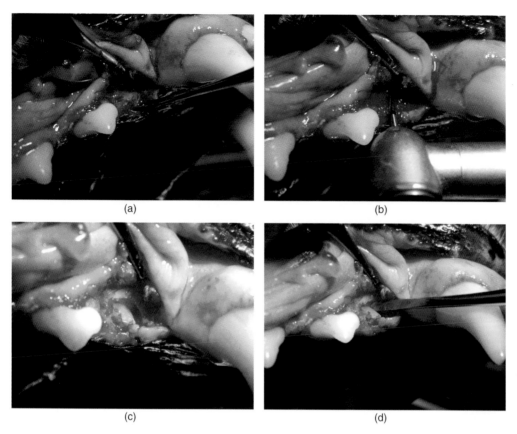

(a)

(b)

(c)

(d)

Figure 11.5 Correct technique for removal of a fractured and retained tooth root of a mandibular first premolar (a) The first step is to create a flap (this author generally prefers an envelope flap) to expose the alveolar bone. (b) Next, a carbide bur (in this case 701) is used to remove buccal alveolar bone to expose the root. (c) After careful bone removal, the root is visible. (d) A small, sharp luxating elevator is used to carefully loosen the root for extraction. Source: Niemiec, Dental Extractions Made Easier, Practical Dental Publishing, used with permission [10].

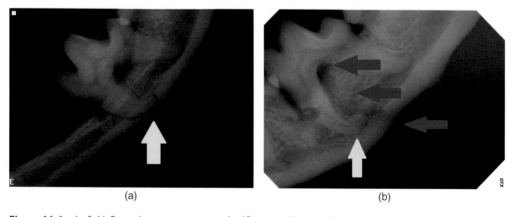

(a)

(b)

Figure 11.6 (a & b) Curved roots can create significant challenges for extraction. Both images are of left mandibular first molars in dogs under 4-kg with marked curves on the mesial root (yellow arrows). In (b) there is also significant periodontal bone loss (red arrows). This makes the extraction of these teeth exceedingly challenging.

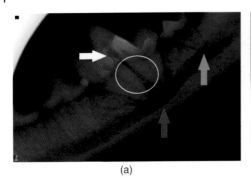
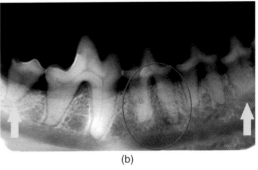

(a)   (b)

Figure 11.7 Root malformations also complicate extraction attempts. (a) Intraoral dental radiograph of a 3.5 kg dog with invergent roots on the mandibular first molar (yellow circle). This makes sectioning and extraction more challenging. In addition, the there is a furcational defect (white arrow) which has created endodontic disease resulting in periapical rarefaction (red arrow). Finally, note that the second molar, which is supposed have two roots, only has one (blue arrow). Therefore, the tooth does not require sectioning and if sectioning was performed, would complicate the extraction. (b) Intraoral dental radiograph of the right mandible of a 2.7 kg dog. The second premolar and second molar, which should have two roots only have one (yellow arrows). Therefore, the tooth does not require sectioning and if sectioning was performed, would complicate the extraction. Also, there is resorption and ankylosis on the fourth premolar (red circle).

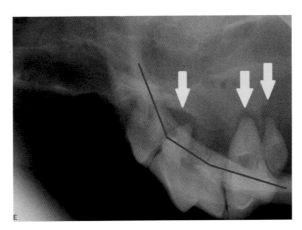

Figure 11.8 Intraoral dental radiograph of the maxillary left of a 10-year-old 1.3 kg dog. The roots of the fourth premolar and molars are right below the globe (the zygomatic arch is delimited by the red line). Extreme care must be taken during extraction of these teeth (especially in brachycephalic breeds) to avoid damaging the eye. These teeth also have advanced periodontal loss and periapical lucency (yellow arrows).

References

1 Lommer, M.J. (2012). Complications of extractions. In: *Oral and Maxillofacial Surgery in Dogs and Cats* (eds. V. FJM and M. Lommner), 153–159. Philadelphia: Elsevier.

2 Gioso, M.A., Shofer, F., Barros, P.S., and Harvery, C.E. Mandible and mandibular first molar tooth measurements in dogs: relationship of radiographic height to body weight. *J. Vet. Dent.* 18 (2): 65–68.

3 Niemiec, B.A. (2008). Case based dental radiology. *Top. Companion Anim. Med.* 24 (1): 4–19.

4 Mulligan, T., Aller, S., and Williams, C. (1998). *Atlas of Canine and Feline Dental Radiography*, 176–183. Trenton, NJ: Veterinary Learning Systems.

5 Hoffmann, T.H. and Gaengler, P. (1996). Clinical and pathomorphological investigation of spontaneously occurring periodontal disease in dogs. *J. Small Anim. Pract.* 37: 471–479.

6 Hamp, S.E., Hamp, M., Olsson, S.E. et al. (1997). Radiography of spontaneous periodontitis in dogs. *J. Periodontal Res.* 32 (7): 589–597.

7 Bauer, A.E., Stella, J., Lemmons, M., and Croney, C.C. (2018). Evaluating the validity and reliability of a visual dental scale for detection of periodontal disease (PD) in non-anesthetized dogs (*Canis familiaris*). *PLoS One* 13 (9): e0203930.

8 Wallis, C., Pesci, I., Colyer, A. et al. (2019 Jun 21). A longitudinal assessment of periodontal disease in Yorkshire terriers. *BMC Vet. Res.* 15 (1): 207.

9 Marretta, S.M. (2012). Maxillofacial fracture complications. In: *Oral and Maxillofacial Surgery in Dogs and Cats* (eds. V. FJM and M. Lommner), 333–342. Philadelphia: Elsevier.

10 Niemiec, B.A. (2013). *Dental Extractions Made Easier*. Tustin, CA: Practical Veterinary Publishing.

11 Niemiec, B.A. (2011). The importance of dental radiology. *Eur. J. Comp. Anim. Pract.* 20 (3): 219–229.

12 Smith, M.M., Smith, E.M., La Croix, N., and Mould, J. (2003). Orbital penetration associated with tooth extraction. *J. Vet. Dent.* 20 (1): 8–17.

Conclusions

Small and toy breed dogs present a completely different clinical picture than do large breeds with regard to periodontal disease and therapy. Periodontal disease has an earlier onset as well as tending to have more severe ramifications than in medium and large breed dogs. Furthermore, small and toy breed dogs are much more prone to other conditions such as persistent deciduous, rotated and crowded, as well as infra-erupted teeth. All of these conditions pose significant health threats and should be treated expediently.

Small dogs are also more at risk for the significant local effects of periodontal disease including pathologic fractures, oronasal fistulas, and orbital inflammation/infection. Finally, their larger proportional gum surface to body mass ratio means that they may be even more subject to the systemic effects. Therefore, we must change our approach and recommend that therapy starts much earlier (before one year of age) and is much more consistent than in larger dogs. This is also true of other at-risk breeds such as Cavalier King Charles Spaniels and Greyhounds.

There are also a number of conditions which are more common in brachycephalic breeds such as impacted as well as rotated and crowded teeth. These conditions should be evaluated and treated as soon as possible. Finally, there are other conditions which appear to have a strong genetic component (e.g. gingival enlargement (GE); canine ulcerative paradental stomatitis (CUPS); and mesio-clused maxillary canines).

Knowledge of these genetic tendencies will help the practitioner to more quickly diagnose these common conditions. Further, it will allow for more accurate and effective discussions with clients, which will improve client compliance with earlier treatment of disease. Finally, if clients are aware of these conditions, they will more likely be more cognizant of the needed therapy.

Breed Predispositions to Dental and Oral Disease in Dogs, First Edition. Edited by Brook A. Niemiec.
© 2021 John Wiley & Sons, Inc. Published 2021 by John Wiley & Sons, Inc.

Index

Note: Page numbers in *italics* refer to figures captions. Page numbers in **bold** refer to tables.